*Reality Check:
Teen Pregnancy
Prevention Strategies
That Work*

Reality Check: Teen Pregnancy Prevention Strategies That Work

Get Real About Teen Pregnancy Campaign

Copyright © 2004 by Get Real About Teen Pregnancy Campaign.

ISBN: Hardcover   1-4134-6667-2
            Softcover   1-4134-6666-4

All rights reserved. No part of this book may be reproduced or transmitted in any form or by any means, electronic or mechanical, including photocopying, recording, or by any information storage and retrieval system, without permission in writing from the copyright owner.

This book was printed in the United States of America.

To order additional copies of this book, contact:
Xlibris Corporation
1-888-795-4274
www.Xlibris.com
Orders@Xlibris.com

TABLE OF CONTENTS

FOREWORD
    Dr. David Satcher,
    16th Surgeon General of the United States

INTRODUCTION 12
    Christi Black and Dawn Wilcox, Program Directors
    "Get Real About Teen Pregnancy"

CHAPTER 1 15
    What the Teens Say
    Sarah Brown, Director
    National Campaign to Prevent Teen Pregnancy

CHAPTER 2 18
    California at the Forefront:
    Building on a History of Wise Investments
    in Teenage Pregnancy Prevention
    Claire Brindis, Dr.P.H., Director
    Center for Reproductive Health Research and Policy
    University of California, San Francisco

CHAPTER 3 27
    Parent Power and More:
    Insights from the National Campaign to
    Prevent Teen Pregnancy
    Sarah Brown, Director
    National Campaign to Prevent Teen Pregnancy

CHAPTER 4 42
Common Design Errors in Teen Pregnancy Prevention Programs: Lessons from Evaluations
Susan Philliber, Ph.D.
Philliber Research Associates

CHAPTER 5 49
Effective Teen Pregnancy Prevention Programs
Douglas Kirby, Ph.D.
ETR Associates

CHAPTER 6 61
Adapted from "Voices of California: A Multi-Cultural Perspective on Teenage Pregnancy"
Debra Nakatomi—Patricia Pérez—Gwendolyn Young
Multicultural Experts

CHAPTER 7 72
Male Involvement & Male Responsibility
Héctor Sánchez-Flores, Senior Research Associate,
Center for Reproductive Health Research and Policy
University of California, San Francisco

CHAPTER 8 80
Every Teen Counts: A Profile of Guillermo Ortega
Dawn Wilcox, Program Director
"Get Real About Teen Pregnancy"

CHAPTER 9 84
Teen Pregnancy Prevention: Politics & Policy
Kathy Kneer, President/CEO
Planned Parenthood Affiliates of California

CHAPTER 10 94
>   *Recent Immigrants and the Role of Parental Involvement in Sexuality Education*
>   Angel Luis Martinez
>   International Sex Educator/Trainer

CHAPTER 11 101
>   *Understanding "Abstinence": Implications for Individuals, Programs and Policies*
>   Cynthia Dailard, Senior Public Policy Associate
>   The Alan Guttmacher Institute

CHAPTER 12 109
>   *Reclaiming Abstinence Education*
>   Tom Klaus, Founder/President
>   Legacy Resource Group

CHAPTER 13 118
>   *Healthy Adolescent Sexuality*
>   Tamara Kreinin, M.H.S.A., President/CEO
>   Sexuality Information and Education Council of the U.S..

CHAPTER 14 129
>   *A Matter of Faith: Reaching Out to Faith Communities for Teenage Pregnancy Prevention*
>   The Rev. Debra W. Haffner, MPH, M.Div., Director
>   Religious Institute on Sexual Morality, Justice, and Healing

CHAPTER 15 139
>   *Adapted from The Sex Lives of Teenagers*
>   Lynn Ponton, M.D.
>   Author, Professor and Psychiatrist

CHAPTER 16 146
> ***Understanding the Concept of***
> ***Sexuality from a Medical Perspective***
> Barbara Staggers, M.D., *Chief of Adolescent Medicine*
> *Children's Hospital and Research Center,*
> *Oakland, California*

CHAPTER 17 154
> ***Lessons from Abroad:***
> ***Strategies to Promote European***
> ***Approaches to Adolescent Sexuality***
> Barbara Huberman, RN, BSN, MeD, *Director*
> *Advocates for Youth*

EPILOGUE 167

ENDNOTES 171

Foreword

By Dr. David Satcher, 16th Surgeon General of the United States

In 2002, when I issued The Surgeon General's Call to Action to Promote Sexual Health and Responsible Sexual Behavior, I knew I was tackling one of the most controversial topics in this country. Every day, our young people are faced with decisions that may impact their sexual health, and yet there is often no place for them to go to get the information and services they so desperately need. We have seen a steady decline in the number of teen births over the past decade. Even so, this year 850,000 teenagers will give birth in the United States. Even more disconcerting are some of the recent reports that have been released detailing sexual trends among low-income black urban youth, who view sex as a transaction and infidelity as a way of life, or the National Campaign to Prevent Teen Pregnancy's report that said one in five teens have sex before their 15th birthday.

While it may sound counterintuitive, the problem of teen pregnancy is largely an adult issue—one that is shaped, determined and perpetuated by the attitudes and behavior of adults and one for which adults must take the initiative in solving. Adolescents must ultimately be responsible for their own behavior, but there are elements of their everyday environment that are largely beyond a teenager's control, including education, economic and family circumstances and availability of health services. At the same time, adults often fail to resolve their own ambivalence about sexuality; this adult ambivalence, in turn, transmits confusing messages about healthy sexuality and contributes to some of the circumstances that allow teen pregnancy to flourish.

At the heart of this issue is a moral dilemma that lies within every adult: how to encourage healthy adolescent sexuality while also protecting our children and keeping them safe. Where the conflict arises is in how much information to share, who's going to share it and when. Adults themselves remain conflicted about sexuality—what's right or what's wrong—and many make their own unhealthy sexual decisions. But it's time to look past our own inner conflicts and consider the health of our young people. Some of them will choose to become sexually active and some will not, but we owe all of them important information that can protect them from disease and unintended pregnancy. Parents have a duty to teach their children their beliefs and values, but they also have a duty to provide them with the necessary, age-appropriate information that allows them to make healthy decisions.

For too long adults have fought over what kind of sexuality education and health services should be available to young people. Too often, the issue for many adults boils down to whether sex among teenagers is an inevitability. This misses a very important point—that teenagers, like all people, possess an innate sexuality whether or not they are actually having sex. This means they will have questions, interests and even desires related to their sexuality. Adults must be ready to provide answers to their questions as well information to protect their health.

The impact of early pregnancy and childbearing is particularly significant for low-income youth. In rural, urban and suburban communities throughout the country, these youth are increasingly marginalized by social, economic and health consequences of teen pregnancy and childbearing. The effect on health status can be particularly serious and long lasting; one-third of pregnant teens receive inadequate prenatal care and babies born to young mothers are more likely to have low birth weights, childhood health problems and hospitalizations than those born to older mothers.

Of equal concern is the rising number of cases of sexually transmitted diseases and infections among teens. More than 19 million new sexually transmitted diseases (STDs) occur every year in the United States, and nine million of those new infections occur in young people between the ages of 15 and 24. In California, more than 30,000 teens were diagnosed with chlamydia in 2000, and with the increasing prevalence of other risky behaviors such as oral and anal sex, there is the possibility of an even greater increase.

Despite these challenges, research tells us that many teenagers have made the decision to take personal responsibility for their behavior and are actively helping their peers prevent pregnancies, avoid STDs and make healthy decisions. In order to continue doing this, they must have informed, educated and dedicated adults assisting them along the way.

Teens need to be valued, respected and expected to act responsibly. Addressing sexual topics with teens in an open and honest manner will have a positive effect on youth and will help instill a sense of respect and responsibility in them. As we stated in the Call to Action, to do this we must continue to promote comprehensive sexuality education for young people, respect diversity in sexual orientation and support families and communities as they work together to create a healthier future for youth.

Dr. David Satcher was named Director of the National Center for Primary Care at the Morehouse School of Medicine in Atlanta, Georgia, in 2002 after serving a four-year tem as the 16th Surgeon General of the United States.

Introduction

By Christi Black and Dawn Wilcox,
Program Directors
"Get Real About Teen Pregnancy"

Many states—California in particular—can be proud of their efforts to reduce teenage pregnancy. Teen birthrates have declined over the last decade by 30 percent in many states, and by 40 percent in California.[1]

Although recent teen birth rate statistics would indicate victory in the effort to reduce teen pregnancy, the future may hold a different story. A study released by the Public Health Institute in 2003 found that because of changing demographics and an increasing teen population, we will likely see a substantial increase in the number of teen births within five years. The potential to have many more teenage parents in the near future is staggering. Therefore, now is the time to identify and continue successful teenage pregnancy prevention strategies.

Reality Check presents a summary of "lessons learned" in the effort to vigorously address teenage pregnancy prevention. The information comes from all over the country, in chapters written by some of the nation's leading experts on the issues of adolescent health, sexuality and pregnancy prevention. Each chapter offers valuable lessons and food for thought to all adults who have any impact on the lives of young people.

Several chapters were authored by experts in California. One of the reasons California has witnessed an impressive decline in teen birthrates is that the state—over three consecutive gubernatorial administrations—made teenage pregnancy prevention a high priority. The state provides significant funding to a variety of programs and endorses comprehensive sexuality education.

Joining the state of California on the front lines in the effort to help adolescents make informed decisions about their reproductive health is The California Wellness Foundation, a private, independent grantmaking organization. In 1995, The California Wellness Foundation established a 10-year, $60-million Teenage Pregnancy Prevention Initiative with the goal of decreasing the rates of teen pregnancy and promoting healthy adolescent sexuality. An important component of the Initiative is the public education program, Get Real About Teen Pregnancy, which educates policy makers, the media and community leaders about effective teenage pregnancy prevention strategies.

Get Real About Teen Pregnancy is pleased to present this compilation of expert perspectives about the issue. We hope that this book provides you with valuable insight and motivates you to help young people make educated, responsible decisions about their health.

As the Get Real slogan states, "Teen pregnancy is also an adult problem. Let's solve it together."

Get Real About Teen Pregnancy is funded by a grant to Ogilvy Public Relations Worldwide by The California Wellness Foundation.

Christi Black is a managing director in the Sacramento office of Ogilvy Public Relations Worldwide. She has served as the program director for the "Get Real About Teen Pregnancy" public education campaign since it launched in 1998.

Dawn Wilcox, APR is a senior vice president in the Los Angeles office of Ogilvy Public Relations Worldwide. She has served as the program manager and campaign spokesperson for "Get Real About Teen Pregnancy" since 1998.

---

[1] Alan Guttmacher Institute, 2003

What the Teens Say

By Sarah Brown, Director
National Campaign to Prevent Teen Pregnancy

A word from teens themselves. The National Campaign has asked teens from all over the country a simple question: If you could give your parents and other important adults advice about how to help you and your friends avoid pregnancy, what would it be? The following tips represent the major themes we heard from teens.[14]

Show us why teen pregnancy is such a bad idea. For instance, let us hear directly from teen parents. Hearing the real story from teen mothers and fathers can make a big difference. Help us understand why teen pregnancy can get in the way of reaching our goals.

Show us what good, responsible relationships look like. We're as influenced by what you do as what you say.

Talk to us honestly about love, sex and relationships. Just because we're young doesn't mean that we can't fall in love or be interested in sex. These feelings are very real and powerful to us. Talk to us about all this (but no lectures, please). If you won't discuss these issues with us, please help us find another adult who will.

Telling us not to have sex is not enough. Explain why you feel that way (if you do) and ask us what we think. Tell us how you felt as a teen but understand that things may be different for us. Discuss emotions, not just health and safety. Listen to us and take our opinions seriously.

Even if we don't ask, we still have questions. How do I know when having sex is the right thing to do? Should I wait until marriage? How far is too far for me or someone my age? How do I handle pressures from my friends? Will having sex make me popular? How do I know if I'm in love? How do I say "no?" If we don't start these conversations, you should.

Whether we're having sex or not, we need to be prepared. We need to know how to avoid pregnancy and sexually transmitted diseases. That means information about abstinence and contraception. We need honest and helpful information from the people we trust most. If we don't get information from you, we are going to get it somewhere else.

If we ask you about sex or contraception, don't assume we are already "doing it." We may just be curious, or we may just want to talk with someone we trust. And don't think giving us information about sex and birth control will encourage us to have sex. We need to know the facts so that we can make good decisions in the future—maybe next week, maybe years from now.

Pay attention to us before we get into trouble. Reward us for doing the right thing—even when it seems like no big deal. Don't shower us with attention only when we do something wrong. Talk with us about our friends, our school, what we're interested in and worried about—even the latest gossip. Come to our games and school things. Show us that you care what is happening in our lives.

Don't leave us alone so much. Sometime we have sex because there's not much else to do. If you can't be home with us after school, make sure we have something to do that we really like, where there are other kids and adults who are comfortable with us. If we're at a party, make sure there is an adult around.

We really care what you think, even if we don't always act like it. Even thought we may look all grown up, we still want your help and advice. But remember, your experiences are not the same as ours, and the choices we face are often different. When we don't end up doing exactly what you tell us to, don't think that you've failed. And don't stop trying.

We hate "the talk" as much as you do. Please don't sit us down for a "sex talk." Instead, start talking with us about sex, love and values when we're young and keep the conversation going as we grow older. Making us feel comfortable and encouraging us to talk and ask questions is important, too—just make sure you listen to the answers.

For us, it's about abstinence and contraception, not either/or. We get it. We know the best way to protect ourselves is not to have sex. But we also need to know about contraception. It seems to us that adults waste an awful lot of time arguing about all this.

Sarah Brown is director of the National Campaign to Prevent Teen Pregnancy, a private, nonprofit initiative. Before co-founding the National Campaign in 1996, Ms. Brown was a senior study director at the Institute of Medicine where she directed numerous projects, mainly in the area of maternal and child health, including a major study on unintended pregnancy.

California at the Forefront: Building on a History of Wise Investments in Teenage Pregnancy Prevention

By Claire Brindis, Dr.P.H., Director
Center for Reproductive Health Research and Policy
University of California, San Francisco

Biology and sociology have combined to create a compelling modern problem, and in California, demographics are compounding the situation. Adolescent pregnancy, always a feature of American life, traditionally has been a private family matter. What makes it a pressing public issue is the changing social environment in which it is occurring and the growing awareness of its serious personal, as well as wider social, educational, health and economic consequences. The age of onset of menstruation has dropped, while the time needed to prepare for full participation in our complex society has lengthened. Given that California has one of the highest rates of teenage pregnancy in the nation, it is imperative that the issue receives high priority in our state's policy, programs and community planning.

While acknowledging the magnitude of the problem, it is important to note that recent data on adolescent pregnancy and childbearing are encouraging. During the 1990s, the teen pregnancy and birthrate declined across the country, in all states, and among all age, racial and ethnic groups. In many cases, these declines have been quite dramatic. Teen pregnancy and abortion rates, for example, are the lowest since they were first measured in the early 1970's.[3]

In 2001, the teen birthrate reached its lowest point in more than six decades,[4] encouraging news although U.S. rates remain substantially higher than other countries, such as England and Canada (twice as high), France (four times as high), and nine times as high as the Netherlands and Japan.[5] In 2001, there were nearly 54,000 births to California mothers under age 20,[6] many of whom were neither emotionally nor economically prepared to raise a child. Of all the births in California that year, approximately one in 10 were to teen mothers.

Teen births vary by age, race/ethnicity and geography. The birthrate is higher for ages 18 and 19 (at 76.6 births per 1,000) than for ages 15 to 17 (4.4 births per 1,000).[7] The rate is higher for Hispanic (86.2 births per 1,000) and African American (53.3 births per 1,000) teens than for white (20.2 births per 1,000) or Asian/Pacific Islander (12.6 births per 1,000) teens ages 15 to 19 (California Department of Health Services n.d.). Teen birthrates are particularly high in the major population centers in the state, including Los Angeles County, San Diego County, the San Francisco Bay Area and the Central Valley.[8]

This profile points to the importance of adolescents' socioeconomic status impacting childbearing. Seventy percent of higher income teens who become pregnant choose to postpone childbearing, whereas lower income teens are more likely to give birth. Poor and low-income teens—who make up approximately 40 percent of the adolescent population—account for 83 percent of teens who give birth and 85 percent of those who become an unmarried parent. There also are marked racial and ethnic differences in the ways teen pregnancy is resolved, perhaps the result of differences in family structure, age at first conception and family size.[9] For example, among whites, being raised in a single-parent family was found to significantly enhance the likelihood of a teen choosing to have a child outside of marriage.[10]

Fortunately, through the past two decades, California has demonstrated a strong commitment to reducing the incidence of teenage pregnancy, and clearly this investment has made a substantial impact. In 1987, the legislature passed Assembly Concurrent Resolution 52 supporting a statewide planning conference to determine the policies, programs and services most needed to both reduce teenage pregnancy and to improve the outcome of pregnancies that do occur, and to develop a comprehensive state plan for reducing adolescent pregnancy. A broad-based coalition of private and public agencies joined forces, recognizing that although policymakers play a vital role, the problem requires active participation of teenagers, parents, religious and community leaders, professionals and the media. Although participants differed in perspectives, fields of expertise and sometimes in their philosophies, they recognized that this is a problem that benefits from multiple and multifaceted approaches. The Strategic Plan for Adolescent Pregnancy and Parenting in California[11] highlighted a number of themes that have shaped the efforts of the state and its partners over the past 15 years, including:

- Promoting the positive development of youth through the active engagement of young people, their families, schools and the broader community,

- Expanding the role of males in sharing responsibility for prevention, reproduction and parenting,
- Strengthening the role of the family in supporting young people,
- Expanding the availability of comprehensive family-life education,
- Expanding access to comprehensive health services to adolescents, including reproductive health care,
- Decreasing the incidence of sexually transmitted infections, including HIV/AIDS,
- Improving educational outcomes for all adolescents,
- Increasing the career planning and job opportunities available to both males and females,
- Expanding the role of schools and the community in preventing adolescent pregnancy and
- Expanding the news media's role in reaching young people with messages of responsible behavior.

These themes were presented within a framework that called for placing the topic of adolescent pregnancy and prevention within a policy agenda, expanding financial investments for strategies that have demonstrated positive outcomes, along with coordinating inter—and intra-agency efforts (for example, both within the state Department of Health, as well as with the state Department of Education and Department of Social Services), as well as state and county agencies directly impacting adolescents.

Since the development of the Strategic Plan, California has demonstrated a strong statewide policy commitment to expanding the types of concurrent efforts aimed at successfully reducing unintended adolescent pregnancy. These efforts represent an understanding of the complexity of the topic, the different segments of the adolescent population and the families that need to be reached (from pre-sexually active adolescents to adolescent parents), the importance of tailoring different strategies to serve each and the importance of comprehensive efforts aimed at both reducing adolescent pregnancy and supporting teenage parents and their families.

These underlying principles reflect a fundamental shift that is occurring in the field, from programs and services that aim to improve the health of teens by focusing on eliminating problems, such as high-risk behaviors, to a new emphasis on considering youth as potential resources in resolving the problem of teenage pregnancy. In the past, programs often blamed youth for their risky sexual behaviors, "without fully acknowledging that adolescent behavior mirrors that of adults and is shaped by their social and cultural environments, including families, communities, schools, media, popular culture and public opinion."[12]

Increasingly, education and services that focus on sexuality and reproductive health are being linked to efforts to strengthen resiliency, the ability of youth to overcome obstacles and build the competencies they need to succeed as adults.[13] Prevention programs now have broader goals for improving academic, social and vocational skills and life prospects. These multifaceted efforts encourage youth to develop connections with their community and to have high expectations for their futures so that they are motivated to delay pregnancy and childbearing until adulthood.[14]

California's successful primary prevention efforts include the following:

- For nearly 30 years, the California Department of Health Services, Office of Family Planning's (DHS-OFP) Information and Education (I & E) projects have provided educational services in a variety of settings, including schools, juvenile justice, foster care and others where youth can be reached with family-life education and teen pregnancy prevention strategies. Parents and other caregivers are supported through health education programs that recognize their role as primary educators.

- The Community Challenge Grant (CCG) Program promoted community-based partnerships that aim to reduce teen and unintended pregnancy and absentee fatherhood, promote responsible parenting and increase the involvement of fathers in the economic, social and emotional development of their children. DHS-OFP has funded more than 130 community-based agencies, school districts, public health agencies, social service agencies and local governments to provide comprehensive family-life education, career and job skills development, mentoring, education and support for parents of teens, and youth development.
- DHS-OFP's Male Involvement Program (MIP) provides local assistance funds to increase the involvement of adolescent and young males in the prevention of unintended pregnancy and fatherhood. The intent of the program is to increase community and individual awareness of the importance of the roles and responsibilities males have in the reduction of teenage pregnancies and to increase the knowledge, skills and motivation of males to assume positive leadership roles in their communities. Interventions provided through the 25 MIP programs include educational sessions; youth leadership development activities; teen theater, conferences and retreats; access to job training and placement; cultural rites-of-passage programs; and peer outreach. (Please note that DHS is undergoing efforts to integrate the aforementioned programs).
- The Teen Pregnancy Prevention Grant Program (TPPGP) was the first effort by the California Department of Education (CDE) to support students in delaying the onset of sexual activity and to reduce teenage pregnancy. For five years (1996-2001), CDE funded school-community partnerships to develop and implement comprehensive prevention programs,

focused on areas with the greatest need. Thirty-seven school districts and county offices of education provided family-life education, youth development, after-school activities, academic support and case management services to students from elementary through high school.

- DHS' Family PACT (Planning, Access, Care and Treatment) Program provides universal access to pregnancy prevention services for eligible women, men and teenagers whose incomes are at or below 200% of the federal poverty level. Family PACT services include client counseling, contraceptive methods, sexually transmitted infection testing and treatment, HIV testing and cancer screening. Family PACT providers include private physicians and physician groups, community clinics, rural health clinics, hospital outpatient departments and health centers. Federal matching dollars, as part of a special Medicaid waiver, are used to pay for services. A cost-benefit analysis found that for every dollar spent on services, the state and the federal government saved an estimated $4.48 in medical and social service costs.[15] The program saved over $512 million in public expenditures that would have been spent on medical care, income support and social services for the mother and for the child born as a result of an unintended pregnancy.
- DHS-OFP's Teen Pregnancy Prevention Media Campaign ("It's Up to Me"), funded for five years, aimed to involve communities and organizations throughout the state. Its predominant message—as shown through public service announcements, billboards, a toll-free referral hot line and a Web site—is that all Californians share responsibility in reducing teen pregnancy. The campaign aimed to mobilize teens, parents, young men and the general public to

help reduce teen pregnancies, encourage adult-teen communication and publicize the availability of Family PACT clinical services.
- The California Wellness Foundation's Teen Pregnancy Prevention Initiative represents a 10-year, privately funded initiative aimed at reaching community groups, organizations and geographic areas with high unmet needs for services, improving the professional training of providers working with youth in a variety of settings, providing scholarship support for promising young people entering the field of teenage pregnancy prevention, supporting researchers and funding a statewide media campaign targeting policymakers and community leaders titled, "Get Real About Teen Pregnancy." As part of the media campaign, special studies have been conducted, including public opinion polling, focus groups and background research, resulting in a series of useful monographs, newspaper ads, a Web site and other communication efforts.[16]

In addition, a number of concurrent strategies are taking place in a variety of communities. Sponsored by community-based organizations, the faith community, schools and others, many focus on youth development and supporting adolescents' pregnancy-free transition into adulthood. These commitments will be important to continue and enhance as California experiences a dramatic increase in the number of people ages 10 to 19 (a 34 percent increase between 1995-2005, in contrast to a 13 percent increase nationally).[17] This represents an approximate increase from 4.5 million to 6 million youth.

This demographic shift has numerous policy implications, particularly because much of the growth is occurring in communities where the need is greatest. Differences in growth by race and ethnicity will result in a new, increasingly diverse portrait of the adolescent population. By 2005, the number of Hispanic youth will grow by 61 percent, Asian youth by 45 percent, African American youth by 22 percent, Caucasian youth by 16 percent and Native American youth by 2 percent. The increase in the numbers of adolescents makes it clear that the issue of adolescent pregnancy will continue to need special consideration. Even at the current teen birthrate, this growth could translate to 59,504 annual births to teens in 2005, an 11 percent increase over the 53,776 births in 2001, solely due to demographic change.

The need to continue a policy and programmatic focus on this issue remains compelling as new cohorts of young people reach this developmental age. We each need to recognize that facing this challenge transcends any one segment of society, as we all face the consequences of teenage pregnancy and childbearing. Thus, it will take a concerted and concentrated effort on each of our parts to continue to impact its successful resolution.

Claire Brindis, Ph.D. is director of the Center for Reproductive Health Policy Research and a professor in the Division of Adolescent Medicine, Department of Pediatrics at the University of California, San Francisco.

Parent Power and More: Insights from the National Campaign to Prevent Teen Pregnancy

By Sarah Brown, Director
National Campaign to Prevent Teen Pregnancy

The topic of this important book, teen pregnancy, should be a top concern of all those interested in social policy, in families, in the life course of young women and in children most of all. The United States has the highest rates of pregnancy, birth and abortion among teens in the fully industrialized world. Even with recent declines, 35 percent of teen girls become pregnant at least once before turning 20, and U.S. taxpayers shoulder at least $7 billion each year in direct costs and lost tax revenues associated with teen pregnancy and childbearing. Both teen mothers and their children face adverse consequences in many areas—health, education, income status and others as well. For example, more than two-thirds of teenage girls who begin their families before age 18 never complete high school. The problems that flow from such limited education—and from a failure to graduate from high school, in particular—have become increasingly serious, in part because of recent economic trends. Jobs that were traditionally available to high school graduates (and that paid a living wage and often came with benefits as well) are rapidly moving outside of the United States, leaving poorly educated Americans, including the majority of teen mothers, even farther behind.[1]

Against this backdrop, the private nonprofit National Campaign to Prevent Teen Pregnancy was organized in 1996 by a diverse group of individuals who had concluded that the problem of teen pregnancy was not receiving the intense national focus that it deserved; that too few Americans understood the central role that teen pregnancy plays in child poverty, out-of-wedlock childbearing and welfare dependence; and that there was merit in both raising the profile of this problem and in pushing hard for solutions. The campaign's mission is to improve the well being of children, youth and families by reducing teen pregnancy; our goal for the nation is to reduce the rate of teen pregnancy by one-third between 1996 and 2005. Recent demographic analyses suggest that the nation may well meet this target.

In our eight years of intense effort, all of us involved in the campaign have learned many lessons, not all of which were even dimly discernable at the beginning. Here are six of them, the last of which—the role of parents in all this—is developed in more depth. The public opinion polling data cited are all from the campaign's annual, nationally representative surveys of adults and teens, unless noted otherwise.[2]

1: Too many parents and other adults in positions of leadership are unwilling to take a strong stand against teen pregnancy.

We have noted a distinct unwillingness among adults—and in the culture generally—to take a clear stand on whether teen pregnancy is or is not OK. Although nine out of ten adults and teens agree that teen pregnancy is a serious problem, fully one-third of adults do not think that the kids in their communities are getting a clear message from the adults in their lives that teen pregnancy is wrong, and fewer than six out of ten teens strongly agree that they are getting a clear message that teen pregnancy is wrong. This may be due to queasiness among adults about taking a stand that has a values component—a sense of not wanting to "impose one's values on another." It also may reflect a popular culture that has become increasingly tolerant of unwed pregnancy and childbearing. Moreover, many parents and adults readily admit that they avoid talking clearly to young people about sex and values because the topic makes them uncomfortable. And some adults are unwilling to take a strong stand against teen pregnancy and childbearing out of concern that they will offend those teens who are already pregnant or parenting or that they might inadvertently stigmatize the children of teen mothers.

But if we can't even say in a simple declarative sentence that teen pregnancy and parenthood is in no one's best interest—that childbearing is for adults (and many would add, "preferably married ones")—how can we be surprised at our high rates? Preventing teen pregnancy is, at a fundamental level, a question of values, standards, social norms and what a given society prescribes as the best pathway from childhood to adult life. It is not just about information and education regarding reproduction. This simple observation has led many to conclude that one of the primary challenges we face if we are to make continued and lasting progress in reducing teen pregnancy is to offer more straight talk to young people—and conversations with them—about the critical need to postpone pregnancy and parenthood until adulthood. Elected officials, teachers, parents and adults generally need to get over their discomfort about taking a clear position on this issue and speaking "early and often" to children about their views and expectations.

2. Strident arguments over which strategy is better—sexual abstinence or contraceptive use—are a recipe for stalemate, and they obscure the more critical issue of motivation. Teens will do neither if they are not highly motivated to avoid pregnancy in the first place.

Far too often, conversations about preventing teen pregnancy disintegrate into acrimonious ideological wrangling over "abstinence versus contraception." In fact, many people working to prevent teen pregnancy at the community level report that this disagreement is one of the most difficult challenges they face in moving ahead. What is striking about this argument, however, is that advocates on both sides of this topic seem to assume that teens are already highly motivated to prevent teen pregnancy and that the only issue in play is deciding the best means to help them do what they already want to do. Yet too many teens themselves make abundantly clear that avoiding teen pregnancy is often of little concern to them, frequently saying "it won't happen to me."

This failure to zero in on motivation flies in the face of both research and common sense. We know that avoiding pregnancy takes will and determination. Remaining abstinent is a tough challenge. Using contraception carefully and consistently is an equally tall order because most contraceptive methods require a constancy of attention and action that is difficult for even married adults to maintain, let alone teenagers. Given this simple reality, research has shown that if a young person is at all ambivalent about the importance of avoiding pregnancy, the risk of becoming pregnant is quite high.[3] Absent strong motivation, the "default" position is too often the riskiest of all: sexual activity with no contraception. When asked about the primary reason teens get pregnant or get someone pregnant, more teens cite a lack of sufficient motivation to avoid pregnancy than any other reason. Older teens (age 15-19) are much more likely than younger ones (age 12-14) to cite a lack of motivation. One-fifth of teens cite the influence of alcohol and drugs, and another fifth cite inattentive parents.[4]

All this suggests that those concerned with preventing teen pregnancy should steer clear of the skirmish that pits abstinence versus contraception. Both work, and both should be deployed. We must fight a two-front war that encourages more abstinence and better contraceptive use among sexually active youth. But more attention also needs to be paid to the first step of all: motivating teens to choose actively not to become pregnant or cause a pregnancy. That is the primary order of business. It often seems that the adults are arguing about which road to take on the journey when many of the teens aren't even in the car.

A final note on all this. Critics of this consensus position often suggest that telling teens not to have sex while also providing them with information about contraception is a confusing "mixed message" that provides no real guidance at all. This strikes most reasonable people as curious. After all, society routinely tells teens not to drink but, if they do, not to drive. How is that different from telling teens not to have sex but, if they do, to use protection? The National Campaign's 2003 public opinion survey shows that neither adults nor teens harbor confusion about this message. Telling teens not to have sex during their middle and high school years, while also providing contraceptive information and services, is described as a clear and specific message by over two-thirds of adults and teens. Moreover, research shows clearly that teaching teens about contraception does not increase the chances that they will have sex.[5]

3. **Effective programs exist and should be expanded, but it is unrealistic to assume that community programs alone will solve this problem.**

Solid research confirms that a variety of community-level and school-based programs can reduce teen pregnancy. Programs ranging from sex and HIV education to those that encourage young people to participate in community service are effective in delaying the onset of sex and pregnancy, increasing the use of contraception and decreasing teen pregnancy. Even virginity pledges, a component of many abstinence programs, can encourage teens to delay sex in certain circumstances, although such teens may be less likely to use contraceptives once they become sexually active.[6] All of this is particularly heartening considering that, until quite recently, precious little was known about what programs might be most effective in preventing teen pregnancy. Moreover, many communities are putting this knowledge to work on the front lines.

But it is unfair to place the entire responsibility for solving the teen pregnancy problem on the backs of such programs. Not all teens are enrolled in programs, not all programs are well-run and even those that ostensibly copy or "replicate" programs found to be effective do not always do as well as the original model. Many community-based programs are small, fragile and often poorly funded. And even the most effective programs may have only modest success.

Programs are also expensive. We estimate, for example, that reaching every teen in the nation who gets pregnant would cost between $3.8 and $21 billion dollars.[7] Partly as a result of these costs, few teens are enrolled in any program at all—nearly nine out of 10 teens we surveyed a few years ago said they had never been enrolled in a teen pregnancy prevention program, and close to seven in 10 adults said they were unaware of any organized effort to prevent teen pregnancy in their community. Of course, it is also true that many teens are enrolled in programs that might not have teen pregnancy prevention as their focus yet may be beneficial in delaying sexual initiation and pregnancy—after-school programs, for instance.

But there is another reason community programs can't do it single-handedly: Teen pregnancy is rooted in broad social phenomena, such as popular culture, the images portrayed in the entertainment media and the values articulated by parents and other adults. Community programs alone cannot counter these very powerful forces. Public and private funders and activists should look hard for ways to influence such broader social forces as a supplement to their more traditional focus on developing and funding local programs. At the National Campaign, we are doing this by working in partnership with the entertainment media to embed constructive messages and ideas into the television shows, Internet sites and magazines that teens and their parents frequent. A message delivered by a favorite character on a soap opera, for instance, can make a lasting impression on a teen or adult. There are undoubtedly other ways to influence the overall culture that should be developed as well. The simple point is that reducing teen pregnancy will likely require a combination of community programs and broader efforts to influence social norms, values and popular culture.

4. Preventing teen pregnancy requires a new commitment to protecting young girls and an increased emphasis on teen pregnancy prevention in the responsible-fatherhood movement.

We have noticed an odd phenomenon. Many organized social sectors have spoken out on the problem of teen pregnancy—child-advocacy groups, health and medical groups, education associations, governors, state legislators, members of Congress and many others. Yet organized women's groups have been essentially silent. We say this not so much to challenge women's groups directly but to underscore the fact that the problem of teen pregnancy is rarely viewed as a broad failure to protect the lives and hearts of young girls and women. This despite the fact that much of the research on factors associated with teen pregnancy can be seen as an indictment of our current culture. Think, for example, about the data on partner differences in age (e.g., young teen girls remain "targets of opportunity" to older guys), statistics on the prevalence of unwanted sex among younger female teens, data on the minuscule number of the fathers of babies born to teen mothers who marry the girl or even stick around, evidence that some portion of teen pregnancy is preceded by child and sexual abuse of girls and the sexualization of girls in the advertising and entertainment worlds especially.

This vulnerability is particularly acute for younger girls. Teen girls who have sex at younger ages are more likely to experience involuntary or unwanted first sex. Also, the younger the teen, the less likely she will be to use contraception. Even among young girls who describe their first sexual intercourse as voluntary, many also describe it as unwanted. Those girls who have had an unwanted sexual experience are more likely to have numerous sexual partners and suffer greater vulnerability to STDs and early pregnancy.[8]

The hundreds of thousands of teen girls who get pregnant each year obviously don't do it alone. For too long, though, this country has relied on classes, lectures and pamphlets targeted primarily to girls as a means for reducing teen pregnancy. Happily, those days seem to be drawing to a close as attention increasingly is being paid to the responsibilities of boys and young men and the critical role that fathers play in the lives of their children. Hundreds of programs designed specifically for teen boys have been established across the country. At last count, 40 states had strategies to prevent unwanted or too-early fatherhood. Almost all are working with young men to define manhood in a way that elevates responsible behavior and values fatherhood. One teen plainly told us, "Having sex doesn't make you a man; waiting until you are ready and responsible does."

From our point of view, this growing emphasis on primary prevention for boys and men—encouraging them not to cause unintended pregnancies in the first place—is a welcome trend. We urge all of those working with teen boys and those working to make sure children have committed and responsible fathers to focus on the importance of delaying fatherhood and avoiding teen pregnancy. They also can help fathers to encourage their own sons and daughters to avoid teen pregnancy.

5. In a diverse country, it is essential to have multiple approaches to preventing teen pregnancy.

We have come to understand that agreement on the best overall strategy to prevent teen pregnancy is not absolutely necessary—only that concerned citizens and leaders take serious, committed action to help teens use their adolescence for education and growing up, not pregnancy and parenthood. Nonetheless, we frequently meet state and local leaders who believe that if they just fight long and hard enough, their neighborhood, county or state will be able to devise an integrated "plan" to prevent teen pregnancy. We have noted this honorable drive among countless state coalitions and local task forces to get it all figured out, all parts working together harmoniously, and all disagreements resolved. Of course, when collaboration is possible it can be a useful thing to do, and there are several state-level coalitions with comprehensive plans that are strong and productive.

But, in truth, we find this devotion to coordinated plans a somewhat quixotic approach. Given the extraordinary and growing diversity of this country, how could the individuals in one community, much less an entire state, always agree on a single set of activities to pursue? Is it realistic to think that deep differences can be eliminated or that single, integrated plans can accommodate all the cultural and religious groups in this country? Rather, we offer a different platform: unity of goal, diversity of means. That is, we "agree to agree" on the goal of reducing teen pregnancy, but, where necessary, we "agree to disagree" about exactly how we will get there.

This platform reflects the country's consensus that pregnancy and parenting are not for the very young but also recognizes that citizens of goodwill have sincere differences about how to achieve this goal. We may make more progress if we urge each concerned group to "tend to its own garden" and spend less energy trying to convince others that their efforts and views are misguided. Some may pursue the remedies of sex education and access to family planning, some may address parent-child communication, some may choose to deliver a strong message of abstinence, some may develop faith-based interventions that stress a particular religious doctrine, and some may emphasize youth development interventions—volunteer service programs, for instance—that may never even mention sex or pregnancy but that nonetheless offer real promise for reducing the likelihood of early sex and pregnancy. In reality, this less-tidy approach may mean that communities present a messy portfolio of uncoordinated activities, some of which may even seem at odds with each other. In our view, that's OK, especially if the alternative is doing nothing much at all.

6. Parents can do much more to help.

Over two decades of research confirms that—whether they believe it or not—parents are an important influence on whether their children become pregnant or cause a pregnancy. Although teen culture often may seem to be little more than a blur of bare midriffs and over-the-top sexual innuendo, parents need to know that—when it comes to young people's decisions about sex—their influence has not been lost to peers and popular culture. They are powerful, and they can use this power in sound, helpful ways.[9]

Our periodic public opinion surveys confirm this view.

Teens cite parents more than any other source as having the most influence over their sexual decision-making. For their part, however, adults believe that peers influence teens' sexual decision-making more than parents. Apparently, parents don't realize how influential they are in this area or how many opportunities they have to shape their children's behavior.

Here are several other key lessons that we've learned: **Children and teens want to hear about sex, love and relationships from parents but often do not.** Parents say they have talked to their children, but the kids report far fewer of such conversations. Parents often report that they don't know what to say given their own checkered pasts and, at times, their current behavior. Parents report that they are confused and overwhelmed by the complicated information that surrounds sex, contraception, and HIV and other STDs. The vast majority of parents believe they should talk to their children about sex but often don't know what to say, how to say it or when to start.

Moreover, adults need to be clear about their own values and communicate them to young people. Children and teens need to know more than just the facts of life. They are influenced by what their parents and other close, caring adults believe and say about love, sex and relationships—as well as by their example.

Research confirms, in particular, that teens who feel connected to their parents are much less likely to engage in any number of risky behaviors, including too-early sex and pregnancy. Overall closeness between parents and their children, shared activities, parental presence in the home and parental caring and concern are all associated with a reduced risk of early sex and/or teen pregnancy. Teens who are close to their parents and feel supported by them are more likely to abstain from sex, wait until they are older to begin having sex, have fewer sexual partners and use contraception more consistently.[10]

Many parents want schools to do more—perhaps because of their own discomfort about talking with their children about sex, love and values. A recent Kaiser Family Foundation survey of students and their parents suggests that parents want schools to do even more than they are already doing in sex education.[11] There is good reason to turn to schools: That's where most teens are; there are sometimes well-trained sex education teachers; peer education can be part of the teaching; and sex-related topics can be included in broader curricula stressing risk reduction, health promotion and disease prevention generally. But there is a downside here. No matter how good the sex education that a particular school might offer, it is unrealistic and perhaps even unwise to think that it can all be left up to schools to put the complex issues of love, sex and relationships in the context that each family prefers. And public schools surely are not the right place to discuss religious teachings about these same issues, even though faith-based values can be a very important part of sexual decision-making.

Here are some additional, parent-related findings from research and from National Campaign's periodic public opinion polling:

More than talk. It is important for parents to discuss sex, love and relationships directly with their children. They need to be clear and candid. Parents should realize, however, that simply talking with their teens about the risks of early sex, for example, without being more deeply involved in their lives and close to them is unlikely to delay first sex, increase contraceptive use or decrease the risk of pregnancy. The overall quality of the relationship appears to be more "protective" than specific conversations about particular sexual issues.

Attitudes and values matter, too. Teens whose parents are clear about the value of abstinence, and/or about the dangers of unprotected intercourse, are more likely to delay first sex or to use contraception. Put another way, parents who provide clear messages about the value of delaying sex have children who are less likely to have intercourse at an early age, and those parents who discuss contraception are also more likely to have children who use contraception when they become sexually active.

Parental supervision. Research supports what common sense suggests—supervising and monitoring teens' behavior makes a difference. Teens whose parents supervise them in an appropriate manner are more likely to be older when they first have sex, to have fewer partners, to use contraception and to be at less risk of pregnancy. It should be noted, however, that "very strict," authoritarian monitoring by parents is associated with a greater risk of teen pregnancy.

Other risky behaviors. The close parent-child relationships that help protect young people from early sex also help to limit other risky behavior, such as violence, substance and alcohol use and school failure. Whether parents are concerned about drinking, drugs, violence, trouble in school, smoking or sex (or all of the above), the best advice is the same—stay closely connected to your teenage sons and daughters.

Parents in the dark. Many parents are not aware that their children have had sex. For example, a recent study confirmed that only about one-third of parents of sexually experienced 14-year-olds believe that their child has had sex. About 50 percent of mothers of 8th to 11th graders are unaware that their sons and daughters had started to have sex.[12]

Dating dangers. Not surprisingly, two of the most powerful risk factors for early sex and pregnancy are close romantic attachments and significant age differences between partners. Romantic relationships between young teens significantly increase the risk of too-early sex. One-on-one dating in the presence of large age differences (three years or more) is also a high-risk proposition. Consider the following information about young adolescents: 13 percent of same-age relationships among those age 12-14 include sexual intercourse. If the partner is two years older, 26 percent of the relationships include sex. If the partner is three or more years older, 33 percent of the relationships include sex.[13] The take-home message is that parents need to discourage early romantic relationships between teens. (We were encouraged recently when, on a nationally televised talk show, a parent bemoaned her 13-year-old daughter's despondency at breaking up with her boyfriend, and the host responded simply, "what is a 13-year-old girl doing with a boyfriend in the first place?")

A national consensus. Most adults share a common-sense approach toward preventing early sexual activity and parenthood: School-age youth should be clearly encouraged not to have sex—both because of important consequences and because sex should be associated with meaning and serious commitment. (In fact, for most Americans, abstinence is not one of several equally attractive options for young people; it is the strongly preferred option). It is also true that even in the face of clear, direct advice to remain abstinent, some young people will not do so. Given this reality, the overwhelming majority of adults also believe that young people should be given information about the benefits and limitations of contraception and provided with appropriate health services, too. In short, public opinion sees a role for both abstinence and contraceptive information and services. It's not either/or, but both.

Give teens credit. Discussing abstinence and contraception at the same time does not confuse teens. The overwhelming weight of scientific evidence suggests that addressing abstinence and contraception does not hasten the onset of sex, increase the frequency of sex or increase the number of sexual partners. And over two-thirds of teens describe messages encouraging abstinence, coupled with information about contraception, as "clear and specific."

In sum, parents who (1) clearly communicate their values and expectations to their children, (2) express their concern and love for them early and often, and (3) exercise supervision—including their child's selection of friends and role models—raise children who are more likely to avoid a host of risky behaviors than parents who do not. The overall strength and closeness of parent/child relationships seems to be the best protection of all.

Sarah Brown is director of the National Campaign to Prevent Teen Pregnancy, a private, nonprofit initiative. Before co-founding the National Campaign in 1996, Ms. Brown was a senior study director at the Institute of Medicine where she directed numerous projects, mainly in the area of maternal and child health, including a major study on unintended pregnancy.

Common Design Errors in Teen Pregnancy Prevention Programs: Lessons from Evaluations

By Susan Philliber, Ph.D.
Philliber Research Associates

After decades of research and evaluation of teen pregnancy prevention programs, it is possible to identify several frequent but avoidable errors in their creation. This chapter outlines some of the most common pitfalls in the design and delivery of teen pregnancy prevention programs and how they can be avoided. The errors and solutions discussed here also apply to programs other than those focused on teen pregnancy, but examples have been chosen to illustrate these challenges in teen pregnancy prevention in particular.

Error 1: Failure to focus on the causal factors

There are only two paths to the prevention of teen pregnancy. Programs can change the sexual behaviors of teens or they can change their contraceptive use patterns. A well-planned teen pregnancy prevention program must clearly articulate how it will affect one of these two general behaviors. Later age at first intercourse, fewer sexual partners and a lower frequency of intercourse illustrate outcomes in the first group. Use of contraception at first or last intercourse, increased frequency of use of contraception and use of more effective methods are examples of contraceptive use outcomes. Sometimes programs fail to make clear how they will affect any of these critical behaviors and thus fail to reduce teen pregnancy.

Another focus problem occurs when programs work on variables so far removed from one of these two critical behaviors that they eventually have little effect. For example, a program might work on decision-making skills among teens. This seems like a rational approach because whether to engage in sexual intercourse is a decision that must be made carefully. Contraceptive use involves a variety of key decisions. Still, if a program concentrates on general decision-making skills, never mentioning or applying the skills to these two critical areas, the program will likely be less effective.

Error 2: Believing that knowledge is closely connected to behavior.

Many teen pregnancy prevention programs are basically educational efforts. While it is reasonable to believe that teens need knowledge about physiology, contraception, reproduction, conception and a whole host of other topics, research teaches us that increased knowledge is not enough. Teens must also have motivation to engage in preventive behaviors, and they fare better when they have support for these behaviors.

A simple assessment of our own behaviors against our knowledge may make this point clear. Most of us know that eating cake is not good for us, that smoking increases our chances of early mortality and that survivability of an automobile accident is much higher when we wear seat belts. Yet eating cake, smoking and failure to buckle up are all too common—behaviors that are contrary to our knowledge about what we "should" do.

This means that while our teen pregnancy prevention programs might have information-giving components, enhanced knowledge alone is unlikely to result in behavior change.

Error 3: Missing the teens that need programs the most.

Teen pregnancy is not distributed randomly in our communities. Instead, it is more common in poorer neighborhoods, in families with more challenges, among children who are not doing well in school, and so on. A well-planned teen pregnancy prevention program should begin with an analysis of where and among whom teen pregnancy rates are highest. Then, program locations and recruitment strategies must be planned to access these places and these young people.

Often, programs work opportunistically, selecting schools where principals will grant access to students or choosing neighborhoods close to their headquarters. This targeting problem gets rationalized by arguing that all teens are at some risk of pregnancy. Indeed, all teens are at some risk, but they are not all at the same risk.

Another way to miss teens most in need is to offer the same interventions to all young people, regardless of risks and needs. This can result in spending lots of time with teens whose risk of teen pregnancy is relatively low comparable to preaching about church attendance to the choir. It also can mean that those in need of strong interventions over time instead receive relatively weak programs.

Error 4: Running a program with low coverage and expecting community impacts.

Sometimes teen pregnancy prevention programs have ambitions to lower the teen pregnancy rate in an entire community, a neighborhood, a county or even a state. Clearly, however, unless enough young people are reached with a planned intervention, these ambitious goals will not be met. It is likewise unrealistic to expect program effects to spread without a planned mechanism to make this happen. For example, some peer education programs assume that knowledgeable teens will tell others what they know about sex and contraception, without creating a realistic plan for this to happen.

Error 5: Offering low intensity, weak interventions.

This is perhaps the most common error in teen pregnancy prevention programs and can occur in a variety of ways. The one-hour lesson on the reproductive system delivered in the ninth grade assembly is an example of such an intervention. No matter how well-delivered, this lesson will not be enough to reduce rates of teen pregnancy.

There are other ways to make interventions relatively weak. The untrained, unmotivated teacher who is uncomfortable with sexuality topics is unlikely to deliver a powerful message. The successful program gets abbreviated by leaving out critical and powerful portions that are more expensive or more controversial. Several lessons or interventions are chosen from 3 or 4 successful programs, creating a miscellaneous set of strategies based on little rationale except program director preference.

Sometimes a poor combination of coverage and intensity

can derail a teen pregnancy prevention program. For example, while media announcements about contraceptive services can reach wide audiences, this is a relatively "light touch" intervention. On the other hand, arranging for a teen to have a complete physical exam, including reproductive health services, is an intense intervention but difficult to deliver to thousands of teens. Program directors need to examine both the coverage and intensity of their planned interventions to get a realistic view of what effects can be expected.

Teen pregnancy is a complex and tenacious problem. A brief, half-hearted or half-baked intervention is quite unlikely to uproot the powerful forces that lead to sexual risk taking and pregnancy. If it were this easy, we would not have the highest rate of teen pregnancy among developed nations.

Error 6: Failure to deliver the program.

There are many programs that are well-planned and include powerful interventions that should work. They fail, however, because they never really get delivered. Eight workshops were planned, but only four were held. The targets were 100 parents, but only 20 could be recruited. Home visits were critical but turned out to be too much of a logistical challenge. Embarrassed teachers skipped all the curriculum chapters that spoke frankly about sex. These are all examples of things planned that were not in fact, delivered. A well-managed program has a good evaluation in place that will sound the alarm quickly when the intervention is not being offered on time or with fidelity.

Some Solutions

There is simply no substitute for good planning before beginning any prevention program. There now exist several succinct and useful summaries of "what works" to prevent teen pregnancy. Every program should begin by reviewing one of these summaries to take advantage of what is already known about what works and what does not. While some program directors believe they cannot afford to adopt a well-researched program, they apparently believe that they can spend money indefinitely on strategies that do not work or on programs whose results are unknown.

A powerful and now popular planning tool is the logic model or theory of change. This tool asks a program to set out its planned strategies, its expected short and longer-term outcomes, and then to reflect on whether this is indeed, a logical plan. Evaluators and program planners use varying versions of this device but perhaps the simplest format is illustrated below:

To reduce rates of teen pregnancy:

WHAT WILL YOU OFFER TO WHOM BY WHEN?	WHAT SHORT-TERM OUTCOMES ARE EXPECTED?	WHAT LONG-TERM OUTCOMES ARE EXPECTED?
For example:	For example:	For example:
A yearlong curriculum on sexuality and reproduction will be offered, coupled with 3 hours per week of volunteer service in the community for all ninth graders in the high school.	Students will increase their knowledge about....	Students will delay onset of sexual intercourse.
	Students will increase their motivation to protect themselves from early pregnancy.	Students who become sexually active will use effective methods of contraception and STD protection.

With such a device, it is possible to check for the errors outlined above. Is the intervention strong enough? Will the program cover enough teens to reduce rates of teen pregnancy in a desired target area? Are ninth graders in the chosen school the appropriate target? Does the model directly focus on the key behaviors related to teen pregnancy?

After planning, another way to avoid these common errors is to create even the simplest tracking and monitoring systems to make sure the program happens. While evaluation of outcomes is of course, most desirable, even a simple system that keeps track of program delivery and student attendance can greatly improve the likelihood of success. If the program is not being offered with fidelity, its chances of success may be diminished. If young people, their parents, or others who are targeted do not attend the program as hoped, its chances of success may be diminished.

Good planning and good monitoring, both with these potential errors in mind, should greatly increase effectiveness of programs whose goal is further reductions in rates of teen pregnancy.

Susan Philliber, Ph.D. is a founder and senior partner at Phillber Research Associates. She has 30 years of experience in evaluation and basic research. With a Ph.D. in sociology and demography, she has been on the faculty at the University of Utah, University of Cincinnati and Columbia University, where she is currently an adjunct professor. She is extensively published and widely recognized for her ability to train program staff and others in evaluation. Dr. Philliber has been the lead evaluator on several national projects in youth development, teen pregnancy, school achievement, community development, juvenile crime prevention and other human services.

Effective Teen Pregnancy Prevention Programs

By Douglas Kirby, Ph.D.
ETR Associates

Despite encouraging progress over the past decade, the overall teen pregnancy rate in the United States remains high. This chapter identifies particular programs that have the potential for reducing teen pregnancy because they have either delayed the initiation of sex, reduced the frequency of sex, reduced the number of partners, increased condom or contraceptive use or actually reduced teen pregnancy itself.

Which Types of Programs Are Effective?

There is substantial evidence that at least four different types of programs can reduce sexual risk-taking among young people and, thereby, prevent teen pregnancy. These four groups of programs were systematically reviewed in "Emerging Answers: Research Findings on Programs to Reduce Teen Pregnancy,[1]" published by the National Campaign to Prevent Teen Pregnancy, and are briefly summarized and updated here.

Sex and HIV Education Programs

The first group of programs includes sex and HIV education programs. These programs have evidence that they delay sex, reduce the frequency of sex, reduce the number of sexual partners, increase condom use or increase contraceptive use. These effects have been demonstrated for as long as one year[2] and for even as long as 31 months.[3] Positive behavioral effects have been observed in programs implemented in a variety of locations, including schools during regular school hours or during weekend hours, community health centers, community detention centers, shelters for runaway youths and residential drug treatment programs.

Some of the evidence supporting these effects is based on rigorous studies with randomized experimental designs.[4] In addition, meta-analyses and reviews of multiple studies also provide positive evidence of impact.[5] Importantly, researchers have identified some of the common characteristics of these effective programs that may contribute to their success.[6]

The curricula of the most effective sex education programs share 10 common characteristics. These programs:

1. Focus on reducing one or more sexual behaviors that lead to unintended pregnancy or HIV/STD infection.
2. Are based on theoretical approaches that have been demonstrated to influence other health-related behaviors. These theories identified specific important sexual risk and protective factors to be targeted.
3. Deliver and consistently reinforce a clear message about abstaining from sexual activity and/or using condoms or other forms of contraception. This appears to be one of the most important characteristics that distinguished effective from ineffective programs.
4. Provide basic, accurate information about the risks of teen sexual activity and about ways to avoid intercourse or methods of protection against pregnancy and STDs.

5. Include activities that address social pressures that influence sexual behavior.
6. Provide examples of and practice with communication, negotiation and refusal skills.
7. Employ teaching methods designed to involve participants and have them personalize the information.
8. Incorporate behavioral goals, teaching methods and materials that are appropriate to the age, sexual experience and culture of the students.
9. Last a sufficient length of time (i.e., more than a few hours).
10. Select teachers or peer leaders who believe in the program and then provide them with adequate training.

Clinic Services

The second group of programs with evidence that they can reduce sexual risk-taking among teens includes clinic services. The research suggests that the counseling and instruction that takes place between a medical provider and a teen patient and the related materials and activities that can support and reinforce that counseling are key to the program's success. Four out of six studies reviewed found positive effects on behavior with brief, modest interventions. Typically these programs increased condom or other contraceptive use for three months to one year. All four of the effective interventions focused on sexual and contraceptive behavior, gave clear messages about abstinence and contraceptive use and included one-on-one consultation about the client's own behavior.

Service Learning Programs

The third group of interventions with evidence of success includes service-learning programs. By definition, service-learning programs include (1) voluntary or unpaid service in the community (e.g., tutoring, working as a teacher's aide, working in nursing or retirement homes, helping out in day care centers or helping fix up parks and recreation areas) and (2) structured time for preparation and reflection before, during and after service (e.g., group discussions, journal writing or papers). Often the service is voluntary, but sometimes it is arranged as part of a class. Often the service is linked to academic instruction in the classroom. Service-learning programs have strong evidence that they reduce actual teen pregnancy rates. Four different studies, three of which evaluated programs in multiple locations, have consistently indicated that service learning reduces either sexual activity or teen pregnancy.[7] The impact on pregnancy appears to last during the academic year in which youth are involved but possibly not beyond.

Comprehensive Programs

The final group of programs includes the Children's Aid Society-Carrera Program. A very rigorous study of the CAS-Carrera Program implemented in six different sites demonstrated that, among girls, it significantly delayed the onset of sex, increased the use of condoms and other effective methods of contraception and reduced pregnancy rates.[8] However, the program did not reduce sexual risk-taking among boys. The CAS-Carrera Program, which is long-term, intensive and expensive, includes the following components: (1) family-life and sex education; (2) individual academic assessment, tutoring, help with homework, preparation for standardized exams and assistance with college entrance; (3) a work-related intervention that includes a job club, stipends, individual bank accounts, employment and career awareness; (4) self-expression through the arts; (5) sports activities and (6) comprehensive health care, including mental health and reproductive health services and contraception. The program also gives a clear message about avoiding unprotected sex and early pregnancy. This is the first and only study to date that includes random assignment, multiple sites and a large sample size that found a positive impact on sexual and contraceptive behavior and pregnancy, among girls for as long as three years.

The studies of these four groups of programs, as well as a few other studies, demonstrate that programs actually can reduce sexual risk-taking and pregnancy among teens. Moreover, the diversity among them shows that there are multiple effective approaches.

Are Programs Effective with a Wide Variety of Groups of Youth and with Higher-Risk Youth?

In addition to knowing that some programs are effective and can be effective in different settings, it is also important to know whether they are effective with diverse groups of young people or only with particular groups. After all, practitioners need to know whether an intervention that was found to be effective with one population of youth is likely to be effective with another. In addition, it is especially important to know whether programs are effective with groups at greater risk of pregnancy.

To help address these issues, Table 1 presents programs that have been found to be effective in different types of communities and with different groups of young people. The examples in the table reveal that the programs identified as having evidence of success are effective across both mixed-income and low-income communities, and across all groups of youth determined by race/ethnicity, gender, age/grade and sexual experience.

As the table shows, a majority of the effective programs have been studied in low-income communities rather than in more middle-class communities or communities with mixed family incomes. This does not mean that programs are not effective in more middle-class or mixed-income communities; in fact, at least six different types of programs have been found to be effective in mixed-income communities. It simply means that people have implemented and evaluated more programs in low-income communities than in middle-class or mixed-income communities. The bottom line is that programs are effective in both low-income and middle-class communities, and the majority have proven effective in low-income communities.

The greatest number of effective programs has been found through evaluation studies involving mixed racial/ethnic groups in which no more than 80 percent of the sample is any single ethnic group. Moreover, these programs also have been found to be effective with each of the three largest ethnic groups (non-Hispanic whites, blacks and Hispanics). The second-greatest number of effective programs has been found to be effective with African American youth, reflecting the large number of programs that have been implemented and evaluated for black youth. Only a couple of programs have been implemented and evaluated for Hispanic youth (making quite clear the need for additional programs and research on programs serving Hispanic youth). Nevertheless, one program that was put in place for multiple ethnic groups was found to be effective for the Hispanic youth within the study. Moreover, other effective programs serving mixed groups of youth were found to be effective with samples that included many Hispanic youth (but not quite 80 percent). Thus, evidence indicates that one or more programs can be effective for all three of the largest ethnic groups.

Similarly, most effective programs were found to be effective in studies that included both males and females, although a few effective programs were designed for only males or only females, and a few programs were effective only for one gender. Programs also have been found to be effective with youth in middle school (typically age 13 and under) and youth in high school (typically age 14 and over). A slightly greater number of effective programs have focused on older youth, but this reflects, in part, the greater number of studies involving older youth.

Finally, programs have been effective with both sexually experienced and inexperienced youth. Some of these programs delayed the initiation of sex and, by definition, were effective with sexually inexperienced youth. Other programs were effective with sexually experienced youth by helping them return to abstinence. Finally, some of the programs increased condom or contraceptive use, sometimes with youth who were sexually experienced before the program and sometimes with youth who initiated sex after the program.

Conclusions

In sum, evaluations support at least four important conclusions:

- Some programs are effective at changing behavior that can in turn reduce teen pregnancy.
- Successful programs represent a variety of different approaches. Thus, different types of agencies working with youth can implement effective programs and make a contribution to reducing teen pregnancy.
- These programs are quite robust—several programs have been found to be effective regardless of the participants' race/ethnicity, gender, age/grade, sexual experience or the income level of their communities. This does not mean that any program can be used with any group—it remains important for practitioners to put programs in place that are appropriate to the characteristics of the youth they are

trying to serve. However, regardless of the group of youth, there are some programs that have been found to be effective with selected groups of young people, and some programs appear to be effective with all of them.
- Programs may be especially effective with higher-risk youth. Many programs have been found to be effective in low-income communities and with black youth who have higher rates of sexual activity. Even more important, analyses of differential effects reveal that some of these programs are more effective with youth who initiate sex early, have unprotected sex or are already teen parents. This is an important finding for policy-makers because these youth are at greatest risk for poor outcomes and have the potential to greatly benefit from such interventions.

How can these positive findings be used to help communities select or design programs to reduce sexual risk-taking and pregnancy? This is not an easy question to answer, and, indeed, several excellent and detailed guides are available to help people design and implement programs.[9]

Many issues need to be considered when choosing what type of programs to put in place. Several of the most important are:

- The actual sexual and contraceptive behavior of teens in the community;
- The values of the community about adolescent abstinence; sexual behavior, and contraceptive use; and childbearing;
- The community's concerns about teen pregnancy only versus concerns about teen pregnancy, STDs and HIV;
- The quality of existing abstinence and sex and HIV/STD education programs in the schools and in other organizations that work with youth in the community;

- The availability of condoms and reproductive health services in the community;
- The extent to which most health care providers address adolescent sexual behavior and how they do so;
- The availability of employment opportunities in the community, the quality of schools, the stability and closeness of families, the monitoring and supervision of youth and the existence of service learning programs and other community programs for youth that may increase connection with responsible adults and
- The resources—both staff resources and monetary resources—available to implement new programs.

With such considerations in mind, there are three strategies that communities should follow to increase the chances that the programs they select or design on their own will actually reduce sexual risk-taking or pregnancy:

1. Implement with fidelity programs demonstrated to be effective with similar populations.
2. Select or design programs that incorporate the key characteristics of programs that have been effective with similar populations (e.g., the ten characteristics of effective sex and HIV education programs).
3. Use logic models to select or design new programs.[10]

When it comes to teen pregnancy, we live in a hopeful time. Declining teen pregnancy and birthrates, combined with a stronger body of research on the risk and protective factors affecting teen sexual risk-taking and on the impact of programs, should increase our confidence to continue building on current success. The challenge will be to integrate what we learn from experience with what we learn from research and to have that pooled knowledge guide our development of more effective programs for youth. Such programs will help young people avoid pregnancy and STDs, make a successful transition to adulthood, become educated and self-sufficient and then become ready to be parents for the next generation.

Douglas Kirby, Ph.D. is a senior research scientist with ETR Associates and is a nationally recognized expert in teen pregnancy prevention research. Dr. Kirby has directed nationwide studies of adolescent sexual behavior, sexuality education programs, school-based clinics, school condom-availability programs and other programs for youth.

Table 1:

Examples of programs that have been found to be effective in delaying sex, increasing contraceptive use or reducing pregnancy by community income level and participants' race/ethnicity, gender, age/grade and sexual experience

	Sex and HIV Education Programs	Clinic Protocols	Service-Learning Programs	CAS Carrera Programs
Community Income Levels				
Communities with Mixed Income	Draw the Line, Reducing the Risk, Safer Choices, Untitled (Klaus et al.)	Untitled (Danielson et al.)	Teen Outreach Program	
Low Income Communities	Postponing Sexual Involvement, Wise Guys, AIDS Prevention for Adolescents in School, Becoming a Responsible Teen, Be Proud Be Responsible, Making a Difference, Making Proud Choices, Healthy Oakland Teens, Untitled (Rotheram-Borus, et al.)	ASSESS, Untitled (Orr, et al.)	Reach for Health with Community Youth Service Learning	CAS Carrera Programs
Race/Ethnicity				
Mixed Race/Ethnicity	Draw the Line, Reducing the Risk, Safer Choices, Teen Talk, Untitled (Klaus et al), Wise Guys, AIDS Prevention for Adolescents in School, Get Real about AIDS, Healthy Oakland Teens, Untitled (Magura et al), Untitled (Rotheram-Borus, et al.)	ASSESS, Untitled (Orr, et al.)	Reach for Health with Community Youth Service Learning, Teen Outreach Program	CAS Carrera Programs

Non-Hispanic White	Reducing the Risk, Safer Choices	Untitled (Danielson et al.), Untitled (Winter et al.)		
Black	Postponing Sexual Involvement, Safer Choices, Becoming a Responsible Teen, Be Proud Be Responsible, Making a Difference, Making Proud Choices			
Hispanic	Safer Choices			
Gender				
Mixed Gender	Reducing the Risk, Safer Choices, AIDS Prevention for Adolescents in School, Becoming a Responsible Teen, Be Proud Be Responsible, Making a Difference, Making Proud Choices, Get Real about AIDS, Healthy Oakland Teens, Untitled (Rotheram-Borus, et al.)	ASSESS	Reach for Health with Community Youth Service Learning	
Male	Draw the Line, McMaster Teen Program, Safer Choices, Teen Talk, Wise Guys, Untitled (Magura et al.)	Untitled (Danielson et al.)		
Female	Reducing the Risk, Safer Choices, Untitled (Klaus et al.)	Untitled (Orr, et al), Untitled (Winter et al.)	Teen Outreach Program	CAS Carrera Programs

Age/Grade				
11-13 Years Old/Grades 6-8	Draw the Line, McMaster Teen Program, Postponing Sexual Involvement, Wise Guys, Making a Difference, Making Proud Choices, Healthy Oakland Teens	ASSESS	Reach for Health with Community Youth Service Learning	
14-19 Years Old/Grades 9-12	Reducing the Risk, Safer Choices, Teen Talk, Untitled (Klaus et al.), AIDS Prevention for Adolescents in School, Becoming a Responsible Teen, Be Proud Be Responsible, Get Real about AIDS, Untitled (Magura et al.), Untitled (Rotheram-Borus, et al.)	ASSESS, Untitled (Orr, et al.), Untitled (Winter et al.)	Teen Outreach Program	CAS Carrera Programs
Sexual Experience at Baseline				
Both Sexually Inexperienced and Experienced	Postponing Sexual Involvement, Reducing the Risk, Safer Choices, Wise Guys, AIDS Prevention for Adolescents in School, Becoming a Responsible Teen, Be Proud Be Responsible, Making a Difference, Making Proud Choices, Get Real about AIDS, Untitled (Magura e		Reach for Health with Community Youth Service Learning, Teen Outreach Program	CAS Carrera Programs
Sexually Inexperienced	Draw the Line, Reducing the Risk, Safer Choices, Untitled (Klaus et al.), Becoming a Responsible Teen, Making a Difference, Making Proud Choices, Healthy Oakland Teens		Reach for Health with Community Youth Service Learning	CAS Carrera Programs
Sexually Experienced	Safer Choices, Teen Talk, Becoming a Responsible Teen, Making a Difference, Making Proud Choices	ASSESS, Untitled (Danielson et al.), Untitled (Orr, et al.), Untitled (Winter et al.)		

Note:

All of these programs met the criteria for inclusion in Emerging Answers and had at least one positive significant behavioral impact. However, some of these programs have much stronger evidence than others that they actually change behavior. See Emerging Answers for more information about which programs have the strongest evidence that they actually change behavior.

Criteria for coding: If 80 percent or more of the sample was a particular race or gender, then it was coded that race or gender. Otherwise it was coded mixed. If a program delayed the initiation of sex, then it was included in the sexually inexperienced category. If it presented separate and significant results for either sexually inexperienced or sexually experienced youth at baseline, then it was coded for the appropriate category. If had effects on both groups, it also was coded both.

Adapted from "Voices of California: A Multi-Cultural Perspective on Teenage Pregnancy"

By Debra Nakatomi, Patricia Pérez and Gwendolyn Young
Multicultural Experts

California's increasingly diverse population poses unique challenges to those involved in teen pregnancy prevention. The state's population, reflecting a myriad of ethnic and cultural backgrounds, with varying degrees of assimilation levels, speaks more than 150 different languages. The concept of "minorities" has taken on a new meaning in California, where the ethnically diverse population boasts a majority of residents. In this state with a population of more than 33 million, nearly 33 percent are Latino, 11 percent are Asian and nearly 7 percent are African American.[1]

Against this backdrop of cultural diversity, government and private funders have dedicated substantial resources to teen pregnancy prevention. The state of California has invested millions of dollars during the past 10 years through intervention and education programs designed to reduce teen pregnancy rates. The state's involvement has been enhanced by teen pregnancy prevention programs and other educational strategies supported by The California Wellness Foundation, the Kaiser Family Foundation and the National Campaign to Prevent Teen Pregnancy, among others. Community health providers and school-based programs funded by state and private resources provide a wealth of information on successful approaches, being responsive to the ethnic and cultural nuances of the communities they serve.

As births to teens continue to drop across the nation, California's teen birthrate recently dipped below the national average for the first time in more than 20 years. However, there were still 45 births per 1,000 teens between the ages of 15 and 19 in 2001, equaling more than 52,966 babies born to teens.[2]

The sense of urgency also increases when birthrates are delineated by ethnicity. The birthrate to Latino teens remains the highest among California's population with 86.2 births per 1,000 teens. African American teens have the next highest birthrate with 53.3 per 1,000 teens, and Asian and Pacific Islanders have the lowest with 12.6 per 1,000 teens.[3] Filipino and Vietnamese represent the second—and third-largest Asian American populations in California, respectively.[4] Births to Vietnamese teens represent nearly 4.5 percent of all teen births, and births to Filipino teens represent 6 percent of all teen births in California.

Although births to teens continue to decline, the rates of sexually transmitted infections (STIs) are climbing among teenagers. It's clear that although pregnancies are being averted, unprotected sexual activity is still occurring. More than 15 million new STIs occur every year in the United States, and one-fourth of those new infections occur in teenagers.[5] In California, more than 30,000 teens were diagnosed with chlamydia in 2000 with rates among African

American teens several times higher than rates for Latinos, Asian and Pacific Islander and Caucasians.[6]

Research has shown that many factors influence the number of teen births among California's diverse populations, including: socioeconomic status of the community or neighborhood in which a young person is raised; cultural norms that dictate behavior patterns, moral codes and values; lack of basic knowledge of reproduction and contraception; and level of access to information and services, specifically health care services.

To fully understand the implications of creating policy and programs that will be effective with a diverse population base, the "Get Real About Teen Pregnancy" public education campaign conducted qualitative and commissioned quantitative research over three years to assess attitudes and develop recommendations on this issue. Two things became clear during this research. First, a "one size fits all" approach is not effective in addressing the needs of ethnic communities. Second, culturally diverse parents share a common belief: They all want what's best for their children, including a future filled with opportunities for success.

Among all ethnic communities, youth development and socioeconomic opportunities are seen as key factors in reducing teen pregnancy. If young people have a sense of hope for the future and a clear sense of how to set and achieve goals, they are less likely to experience an unplanned pregnancy or to choose early parenting. Likewise, they are more likely to take steps to prevent pregnancy.

Regardless of ethnicity, the influence of parents or other important adults in a child's life is seen as important to reducing the risk factors of early sexual involvement or teen pregnancy. In ethnic communities, however, although parents agree that their children need to be informed/educated about sex, they express concern about their own ability to be effective in sharing this information with their children.

Framing the Issue in the African American Community

California's African American population is concentrated primarily in Los Angeles, San Diego, Fresno and Oakland. Teen birthrates are particularly high in these major population centers.[7] According to the U.S. Department of Health and Human Services, African American youth are significantly more likely than their white and Latino counterparts to become sexually active before the age of 13. However, of those teens who report being sexually active, 70 percent reported condom use.[8]

From a cultural perspective, opinions about teen pregnancy and teen pregnancy prevention are as diverse as the African American community itself. There are differences of opinion based on region, level of existing involvement in teen pregnancy prevention programs and levels of understanding about the environment in which teens live. However, some observations were made while conducting this research.

First and foremost, many African Americans believe that education and community involvement are critical strategies that must be employed to prevent teen pregnancy. Yet when asked if there are specific cultural nuances that affect teen pregnancy or development of solutions, many of those we interviewed felt that there isn't an overwhelming cultural aspect; rather it is a socioeconomic phenomenon.

African American adults tend to support abstinence-only messages directed to teens, yet they want teens to have solid information about contraception in case they become sexually active. There is acknowledgement that this issue is complex and does not lend itself to a one-size-fits-all approach, which calls for additional information to enhance the basic "don't have sex" theme. One primary reason for this is the overwhelming research data indicating that African American youth become sexually active at an earlier age than their counterparts, and that sexually active young people who do not use contraception are likely to experience pregnancy within the first year of having sex.

African American adults expressed concern that African American communities and families send mixed messages to youth. On one hand, adults say they don't want their teens having babies, yet when the baby is born, it is rightfully welcomed into homes and communities. Often the young mother is showered with more attention than the young girl had ever previously experienced. The resulting mixed messages add to the confusion about whether or not teen pregnancy is supported or not supported, acceptable behavior or unacceptable behavior within the African American community structure.

African American adults reported they believe that the most critical issues concerning teen pregnancy are lost or delayed educational opportunities and the economic hardships for the family and the community. They agreed that African American teens respond well to role models who help them make a variety of decisions about how to have a healthy life and successful future. Adults also agreed that the best thing they can do is help teens develop goals and skills to have a successful future, which is good incentive to prevent early pregnancy.

Many adults lamented the decline in African American-dominant neighborhoods where adults look after the welfare of each other's children and have a positive influence in young people's lives.

The faith community plays a pivotal role in teen pregnancy prevention efforts. To address this, it was essential to convene a faith leader-focused dialogue. The faith leaders who participated agreed they must resume their role as cultural leaders and combat the negative media influences on youth, give youth and adults facts and statistics that are relevant to them, encourage adults (including other religious leaders) to "practice what they preach," begin sexuality education prior to the teen years, address the feeling of hopelessness among African American youth and make a commitment to continuing interfaith dialogue.

The African American stakeholders interviewed reported that all policymakers should view teens as the pivot point for California's future. As such, stakeholders expect leaders to develop programmatic solutions and policies that remove barriers, such as teen pregnancy, that hinder young adults' opportunities for success.

Framing the Issue in the Asian American and Pacific Islander Communities

Asian American and Pacific Islanders (AAPI) constitute a large, heterogeneous population that includes members of 34 ethnic groups differing in language, culture and length of residence in the United States. Opinions about teen pregnancy and prevention strategies are as diverse as the groups themselves. California has the greatest number of AAPIs nationwide, accounting for 36.5 percent of all Asian Americans and 29.3 percent of all Pacific Islanders in the United States.[9]

Teen pregnancy among AAPIs largely has been ignored by both service providers and members of the community because of the misperception that they are far less susceptible than the general population. In sharp contrast to this stereotype, research has shown that when teen birthrates are disaggregated by ethnic subgroup, some AAPIs have the highest rates relative to their population size among all ethnic communities in California.[10]

The research conducted by Get Real looked at AAPI ethnic groups with the highest percentage of teen births and did not include research conducted with Chinese, Korean and Japanese populations because they have some of the lowest rates in California.[11]

Recent immigrant parents are at a huge disadvantage for

understanding the pressures their teens are experiencing. The generation gap compounds the cultural divide that accounts for the tremendous differences between values and traditions in their country of origin versus those in the United States. This dynamic contributes to the pressures experienced by youth who don't have a clear identity as either Asian or American. The conflict between tradition and assimilation makes it difficult for parents to exert control over the behavior of their children. This is further compounded by situations of role-reversal when the children become translators for their limited-English-speaking elders.

Asian American females, in particular, face a conflict between their educational and professional aspirations and traditional women's revered role as wife and mother. Second—and third-generation families that have assimilated tend to have a less-traditional outlook than more-recent immigrants.

Many AAPI adults refuse to talk about sexuality with their children because of embarrassment or shame, and many believe it will only encourage teenage sexual activity. Parents generally acknowledge the reality of teen pregnancy, even though some may have difficulty recognizing their own child's risk. When a teen does become pregnant, the issue is treated as a private family matter rather than a community concern.

In certain communities, teen pregnancy brings tremendous shame to the family and, in some instances, is cause for being disowned.

Among other ethnic groups, particularly Hmong and Mien, being pregnant at the age of 16 is more a cultural norm than a stigma. Frequently when teens do become pregnant, families encourage them to get married and will assist the young couple with raising the child.

Early marriage is a tradition in the Hmong and Laotian communities, and teen pregnancy is a normal outcome of this practice. However, the economic and emotional demands of raising a family are bringing about change in this practice.

Risky sexual behavior is tied to involvement in the gang culture for some AAPI youth, including Cambodian, Filipino, Laotian and Vietnamese. Teen pregnancy is one byproduct of the gang initiation ritual for girls. It also serves as the only respectable (and safe) way for members to leave a gang.

Many Asian adults—of all cultures—feel the pressure of being members of minority communities that are constantly under scrutiny by the mainstream. When teen pregnancy is presented as a social issue in context of the larger community, it takes on additional meaning and has broader implications.

Any approaches to teen pregnancy prevention must take into account the ethnic characteristics and tremendous variations among the AAPI subgroups.

Framing the Issue—Latino Community

Latinos have become the most impacted group in regards to teen pregnancy in California. More than half of Latino teens report having sex and placing themselves at risk of becoming teen parents.[12] Although teen pregnancy rates are decreasing statewide, they are decreasing at a much slower rate for Latinos. In 2000, there were 36,892 births to Latino teens in California, representing 67 percent of all teen births in the state.[13] Although the overall rate of teen births has decreased in the Caucasian and African American communities by more than 40 percent, among Latino teens the rate of decline has only been 31 percent.[14]

There are many factors that contribute to high Latino teen pregnancy rates. This is a community that is averse to discussing sexuality and accepting the reality of teenagers' sexual activity. Rather than openly discussing the issue with their children, Latino parents often rely on public schools to educate their children about sex and reproductive health. Although Latinos are the fastest—growing and youngest major racial/ethnic group in the United States, they are also more likely to live at or below poverty levels and have a higher high school dropout rate than any other ethnic/racial group in the country.[15] Teens with limited educational or career goals are more likely to be young parents.

Latino youth engage in unprotected sex for a variety of reasons. These reasons range from difficulty accessing pregnancy prevention programs because of language barriers and fear among undocumented immigrants of using public services, to the desire to start a family or to attain the status and respect that the Latino culture confers on parents.

The level of acculturation among residents also plays a role in teen pregnancy prevention issues, attitudes and behavior. A large majority of California's Latino population emigrated, particularly from Mexico. This is especially important when considering that "Mexican-origin teens have the highest birthrate of all Latino groups (112 per 1,000)."[16]

Family support and community interaction is very important to Latinos, making it especially important to address this issue from a community perspective. Community pressures are more influential to personal behavior among Latinos than the Catholic Church, as it is commonly assumed. Teens tend to make decisions independent of what the church may condone, but they are seriously concerned about not alienating their immediate community, including family members or close family friends.

There is a strong desire among Latino parents and community leaders for teens to delay sexual activity and pregnancy in favor of pursuing education and career opportunities. However, once a young Latino couple has a baby, the family and community support structure tends to welcome the infant with open arms and showers the young mother with abundant attention. This presents a perceived "double standard" within the Latino community that parents and community leaders acknowledge.

"Adolescence is often a turning point in people's lives and a time when choices have potentially long-term consequences. This is particularly true in the area of sexual behavior. The difficulties of navigating through this life stage, compounded by the challenges of navigating two cultures, can make the teen years especially perilous for young Latinos. Having few economic and/or social resources on which to rely further exacerbates these challenges and increases the odds of negative outcomes. A better understanding of how acculturation influences the choices that young Latinos make is imperative if we are to shape programs, policies and interventions that are to be effective in attaining such goals as a reduction in teen pregnancy and STIs." [17]

As California continues to grow and the population becomes even more diverse, it is important to take cultural and ethnic backgrounds into consideration when creating, supporting or implementing teen pregnancy prevention efforts. Programs and outreach must be designed for the populations they serve. Funding must be allocated not only by geographic and statistical considerations, such as total population numbers and birthrates within the population, but also by cultural and ethnic considerations.

The Latino health, education and social service leaders interviewed for this report recommend:

- Respected adults in each community, regardless of the level of professional involvement with teens, must be recruited to assist parents and community-based organizations in understanding the impact of teen pregnancy in their community and learn how to help teens avoid unplanned pregnancies and infections.
- Schools and community-based organizations should make comprehensive sexuality education classes available to adults and teenagers in the primary languages specific to each neighborhood.
- Same-ethnicity health care specialists, psychologists, teachers and other officials need to be included in workshops and community forums where parents and other adults who work with teens can learn how to

help the young people avoid unplanned pregnancy and prevent sexually transmitted infections.

- "Nontraditional" community partners must be included in the effort to help educate teens about reproductive health and motivate them to make informed decisions about their lives. This means including churches, local media, recreation programs, law enforcement agencies, job training centers and businesses in the community effort to help teens realize their future potential by preventing unplanned pregnancies.

Gwendolyn W. Young is president of Young Communications Group, Inc., a strategic communications/public relations agency specializing in social marketing and developing campaigns that reach the emerging majority populations, African Americans, women and people over 50.

Debra Nakatomi is president of Nakatomi & Associates, Inc., a firm specializing in health promotion, education and awareness, social advocacy and community engagement. Her firm has developed innovative programs to address disparities of access for diverse communities while promoting community participation, leadership and media advocacy.

Patricia Pérez is a partner at Valencia, Pérez & Echeveste, the nation's leading independent Latino public relations agency. VPE was established to serve the needs of corporate, governmental and nonprofit entities seeking to reach the growing U.S. Latino market through culturally relevant relationship-building techniques.

Male Involvement & Male Responsibility

**By Héctor Sánchez-Flores,
Senior Research Associate,
Center for Reproductive Health Research and Policy
University of California, San Francisco**

Teen pregnancy prevention efforts historically were developed to assist young women in avoiding early unintended pregnancy. This focus was established because females who became pregnant were impacted directly, immediately and bore the overwhelming weight of raising a child, often with limited and sparse financial or emotional support from the child's father. The result was that programs were developed for young women, and young men were rarely a priority of program implementers.

In 1995, the California Office of Family Planning implemented the current generation of Male Involvement Programs (MIP). The Male Involvement Initiative was a demonstration project that directed resources to local organizations so they could develop and implement teen pregnancy prevention and male responsibility efforts directly toward young men. The result of this focused funding was that a new group was introduced to the established advocates of teen pregnancy prevention.

The topics that MIP have deemed essential include the following:

- Comprehensive and medically accurate sexual health information (including abstinence);
- Knowing where reproductive health resources exist in your community and knowing how to effectively access them;
- Defining and nurturing healthy and respectful relationships;
- Exploring the desired attributes of a partner or spouse;
- Determining whether a young man desires children, how many and when:
- Understanding how manhood is defined by a person, peer group, family and community;
- Developing and using your talents to make positive contributions to your family and community and
- Creating and/or strengthening leadership skills to serve as an advocate for yourself, your family and community.

However, there had been a previous generation of male involvement programs in the 1970's. The documentation of the lessons learned was scant, and there was very little insight that could be obtained to inform the newly established MIP. What can be gleaned from the limited documentation was that the original effort had as a significant goal to assist men to become better supporters of their partners' reproductive health desires. It is safe to imply that men were seen primarily as critical intermediaries to improving women's reproductive health.

The group of projects funded to conduct MIP efforts and reach males quickly adopted a distinct perspective. These program directors knew that young men needed education and prevention strategies that were developed with a male's needs in mind, provided information that was adapted to a male mindset and bridged the gap between prevention and clinical services. Secondly, a more holistic approach was adopted so that larger themes could be included in prevention efforts, such as the exploration and understanding of responsible manhood and reminding young men that they needed this information for their own benefit.

Because young men were considered a new audience for teen pregnancy prevention efforts, there was much to learn. Projects looked to other prevention efforts that had historically served young men, primarily gang and alcohol-drug prevention efforts. The programs discovered that programmers viewed their clientele as walking risk factors making the interventions one dimensional, i.e. don't join gangs because they are dangerous to you and your community, drugs are physically harmful and physically damaging, etc. The unspoken paradigm among local MIP programs and staff was that their interventions would be asset-based, thus capitalizing on the strengths their clients already possessed and then building new skills.

Even with an asset-based approach, the fact remained that programs needed to reach young men. Initially it was believed that incentives or "hooks" would be necessary for programs to conduct effective outreach to reach the number of young men required by the funding source. The logic behind this thinking was that participants would need more than just information to attend and persist in teen pregnancy prevention programs. However the first lesson that participants taught programs was that engagement was preferred over outreach and incentives.

The clearest example of this lesson occurred in San Francisco, where the MIP project was serving a population that had already fathered a child and was seen as being at high risk of fathering a second child very quickly. These young men were enticed to participate with the agreement that once they completed the program they would receive a pair of highly desired and expensive basketball shoes. The program included the topics of responsible fatherhood, reproductive health and contraceptive information and provided the participants a venue to connect with other young men who wanted to improve their fathering skills and their own lives. At the conclusion of the program, the young men requested that the program redirect the funds intended for their shoes to the purchase of items that would benefit their children directly such as diapers and other essentials. The program succeeded in engaging the young fathers in the discussion and learning process so well that they looked beyond their own desire to have highly prized basketball shoes and attempted to meet the needs of their children.

Staff in other areas of California learned similar lessons early in the implementation of MIP efforts. The result was that incentives were de-emphasized, and greater attention was placed on the program content and how staff could make the topic of teen pregnancy resonate with young men in their community. Years later, it is not uncommon to meet young men who have participated in their local MIP project for more than a year, and when asked why they continue to attend, they indicate that there is a connection with the topics addressed, the staff who deliver the program and the project goals themselves. Many participants have gone on to become peer educators, staff educators and program coordinators.

MIP projects were funded to focus prevention efforts in communities considered "hot spots" for teen pregnancy. However, in addition to having higher than average rates of teen pregnancy, these communities also had other markers that placed young men at risk for a multitude of behaviors that can contribute to fathering a child too early and without intention, behaviors such as school attrition, influence of gangs and community violence, experimentation and use of alcohol and illicit drugs.

Initially, most programs took the path of "least community resistance" by serving the needs of young men who were already fathers, or young men who were in alternative school or juvenile detention settings. In most communities, these populations were seen as requiring interventions over prevention but also in great need of the information that MIP was offering. Program staff learned to serve a population that many other teen pregnancy prevention efforts avoided because they were seen as uncooperative or disinterested in the topics of conventional teen pregnancy prevention providers. Over time, MIP projects became adept at designing interventions that actively engaged participants. Teachers, administrators and juvenile justice professionals began to take notice and ask questions.

The history that some alternative schools and detention facilities had with teen pregnancy prevention programs was that programs offered one-time education classes that were included in existing life-skills or health classes. In contrast, MIP programs offered a series of classes that ranged from six to 15 weeks. Skepticism existed among many that young men would be able and willing to sit through the series of classes. At one site, local probation officials thought that the program staff was colluding with the wards in their custody and bad mouthing the detention staff as a way to ingratiate participants with the program. Because why else would participants persist in the program? When detention staff sat in on the education classes, they discovered that the MIP was using teaching strategies that allowed young men to freely ask questions about the topic of the day without being talked down to and allowed participants to openly discuss the realities that they confront in trying to act responsibly or concerns they confront when they failed to act responsibly. The staff helped young men connect topics such as fatherlessness or relationships with their current circumstances and whether it was their desire to father or parent in a similar manner.

Currently, MIP education efforts are offered in more diverse locales that include community youth centers and considered to be mainstream. The entrée to these venues was as a direct result of the success MIP staff enjoyed in reaching those considered hard to reach, coupled with communities realizing that teen pregnancy prevention, as opposed to intervention, developed specifically for males was necessary for a broader group of young men.

Male involvement and male responsibility are seen as synonymous. However, if our priority is to provide young men with the information and skills they need to responsibly navigate their sexual and reproductive health, male involvement is required. Male responsibility is a highly desired behavioral outcome that we urge young men to incorporate on many dimensions in their daily lives.

Within these general categories, programs introduced and addressed topics such as HIV/AIDS awareness, contraception and consistent condom use, the effects of alcohol and drugs on decision-making, community and relationship violence, parental communication and understanding your personal and familial values.

However, some questions arise when the topics described above are fully understood. The questions each parent and community must answer include: What age should young men receive prevention education or intervention services, and who will teach young men about these topics? This conflict of when and who will engage males on these topics has a profound impact on how young men understand and live their sexual and reproductive lives. Especially because other inputs such as popular music, television and films that influence their sexual attitudes are unrelenting. The indecision among adults does not delay the physical and emotional maturation process of boys and young men.

Young men understand that society and the media send them and their female counterparts conflicting messages about gender roles, accepted behaviors and significant to teen pregnancy prevention, what sexual and reproductive health means to them. The sexual health of young men easily can be overlooked because they lack one common primary moment in their lives that signifies a reproductive transition similar to the onset of menses for a young women. As a result, parents and other significant adults struggle to determine when they should begin to address sexual and reproductive topics with young men, fearing that if done too early these conversations will create ideas that were previously unexplored or unknown.

MIPs have effectively worked to confront these issues and advocate for broader inclusion of males in the reproductive and sexual health arena. Projects have accomplished this through generating a greater awareness of the needs of young men through their participation in local coalitions, statewide networks and national task forces.

Although projects received resources to fund prevention education services, staff realized that their clients needed a myriad of other services to successfully navigate from adolescence to adulthood. Consequently, partnerships were established with youth employment services to assist MIP participants with job readiness and employment seeking. Projects linked with medical and reproductive health service providers to build their capacity to attract and effectively serve the sexual health needs of young men. MIP agencies connected with social service providers to identify gaps in community services that can hinder a young man's success in getting off probation or re-entering school. And finally, many staff established lines of communication with the parents of program participants so that parents knew the MIP educators and trusted them as a responsible resource influencing their son.

Male Involvement Programs understand they share common goals with other teen pregnancy prevention efforts. Among the common general goals are reducing teen motherhood and fatherhood, increasing the level of medically accurate information that is shared with males and females, assisting young people in developing a common language so that they can discuss reproductive health, sexual limits and desires and helping young people examine the double standards that exist and negatively affect all young people in insidious and overt ways.

Finally, male involvement includes the provision of medical messages that promotes the maintenance of good general health and the offering of comprehensive clinical services that includes reproductive health services. Young men must be provided meaningful access to clinical services that meet their needs and include: general health screening, respectful consultations that acknowledge the age and level of knowledge the young male patient possesses and tailored medical screenings derived from a young man's experience and life practices based on accepted medical protocols.

Ultimately, the success of MIP should be measured through the respectful interaction between two young people when they are alone, communicating their sexual limits and desires, each respecting the other's right to exist in a noncoercive relationship and relieved of any outside pressure to engage in having sexual intercourse while using a common language that promotes mutual responsibility and healthy behaviors.

Héctor Sánchez-Flores is a senior research associate at the Center for Reproductive Health Research & Policy, Institute for Health Policy Studies at the University of California, San Francisco. Mr. Sánchez—Flores was also a program liaison for the Office of Family Planning-funded Male Involvement Programs, which received national attention for their innovative approaches to teen pregnancy prevention.

Every Teen Counts: A Profile of Guillermo Ortega

By Dawn Wilcox, Program Director
"Get Real About Teen Pregnancy"

"We are not kids today. We are not those people. We are real. We care about this issue. This is our story."
Some might say Guillermo Ortega is a success story or that he's made a lasting impact on all those he's met; others will say outright he's the reason teen pregnancy rates dropped in his community. Guillermo would never take credit for any of those things. In fact, if his mother hadn't dragged him to a community parent-teen meeting when he was 16, he probably wouldn't be attending a state university on a full scholarship.

"I was born in Mexico and lived there until I was 8 years old," Guillermo explained. "I was a quiet kid without a lot of friends, but I did well in math and classes like that. I didn't talk much, as my speech wasn't good, and I got picked on a lot."

After moving to the United States, he started taking classes at the public school and soon was speaking English as well as, if not better than Spanish. Language barriers in his family were tough to deal with, especially as a young child who just wanted to make friends, go to school and play.

Guillermo began his work in teen pregnancy prevention at the Vista Community Clinic in Oceanside, Calif., as a teen assistant on the Every Teen Counts project, a community-based teen pregnancy prevention program funded by The California Wellness Foundation. He was promoted to peer provider when their teen clinic opened and eventually moved up to outreach specialist, a position that allowed him to speak in local schools and agencies that work with troubled youth.

"Every Teen Counts used to have parent-teen meetings every week that my mom would go to," Guillermo said. "One day, my mom invited me to come along so we went together. At first, it felt like church, like I was being forced to go, but then I kept going and started to enjoy it. Personally, I think she wanted me to go so we wouldn't get in arguments any more."

After he attended several meetings, the staff noticed Guillermo's weekly commitment so they started giving him volunteer projects. Soon after, they offered him the job of teen assistant in the recently opened teen clinic. At first, he felt awkward because some of the teens who came into the clinic were older than him. It didn't take him much time to complete the necessary training, and he eventually began conducting screenings with new patients, working at the front desk and processing lab work.

"Since I was bilingual and willing to answer any question a teen might have, I started to get more inquiries than I could handle. Eventually, I was able to train some of the other teen assistants so that I could focus on one-on-one interaction with the teens that came into the clinic. There was this one girl who came into the clinic two or three times a week to talk with the counselors and eventually to get condoms. One of the female counselors pulled her aside to talk with her to see if she was planning to have sex. Turns out she wasn't, but she was considering it and just wanted to be prepared. If the teen clinic wasn't there, she could have ended up pregnant or with a sexually transmitted disease."

Eventually, Guillermo was working 30 hours a week at the teen clinic in addition to taking classes at the local junior college and playing soccer. His experience inspired him to pursue a career in nursing.

"I want to be able to work directly with patients. I love the health field, and because I speak both English and Spanish, I know I can help a lot of people, especially those in need of health care in my community. There aren't a lot of Spanish-speaking nurses, especially ones that are male, so I want to fill that need."

Guillermo applied for and won a scholarship through the Youth for Adolescent Pregnancy Prevention Leadership Recognition Program that will fund five years of schooling in a health-related field. He chose to take his scholarship and attend Fresno State University, where he continues to study nursing. He hopes to start playing soccer again even while juggling a full load of classes and a part-time job.

He wants policy-makers to know that teens aren't ignorant and that they do know about sex, but a lot of things are misunderstood. He believes teens don't get pregnant because they're dumb or just don't understand—it's that the education and information they need isn't always available. Not all teens have the access they need and deserve—policy-makers can help by making sure every neighborhood and every community has programs and services for teens.

"Adults should have to go through the same type of training I completed to be a peer educator, and it would be even better if parents and teens would do the training together. Parents need to start early by answering their children's questions as soon as they're asked. I'd ask my mom questions like, 'How are babies born?' and she'd ask me, 'Why do you want to know?' and I'd say, 'Because I'm 16!'"

Guillermo is passionate about many things and has worked hard to make a difference in the health and lives of other teens. He believes that adults need to not be so judgmental of young people but should spend time getting to know them and finding out what they're passionate about. He likes to remind adults that image isn't a true measure of personality or even the ability to succeed. He credits his parents for loving him unconditionally and for working hard to provide him with not only necessities, but also opportunities.

"If it wasn't for my mom introducing me to Every Teen Counts and then having people there who saw the potential in me, who knows what I'd be doing now? But what I do know is that every teen does count."

Guillermo Ortega is an undergraduate student at Fresno State University in Fresno, California, working toward a Bachelor of Science degree in nursing. Since age 15, Mr. Ortega has volunteered and worked in various positions including teen assistant, peer provider and outreach specialist for Vista Community Clinic and the Every Teen Counts teen pregnancy prevention project in Oceanside, California.

Teen Pregnancy Prevention: Politics & Policy

By Kathy Kneer, President/CEO
Planned Parenthood Affiliates of California

"We know the best way to protect ourselves is not to have sex. But we also need to know about contraception. It seems to us that adults waste an awful lot of time arguing about all this." (Excerpt: What Teens Want Parents to Know.)

To best understand the politics surrounding teen pregnancy prevention in the 21st century, one needs to look to history because, "Those who cannot remember the past are condemned to repeat it," George Santayana, (1865-1952).

The current political controversy surrounding the federal "abstinence wars" has its beginnings as far back as 1870. Abstinence for birth control within marriage was the agenda of the Voluntary Motherhood Movement that was promoted in the United States during the 1870's by feminists such as Elizabeth Cady Stanton and Susan B. Anthony. Suffragists believed that husbands as well as wives should just do without sex altogether in order to control the size of their families.[1]

Abstinence for birth control among married women, however, led to even greater reliance on prostitution by married men, which in turn, led to epidemics of sexually transmitted infections by the turn of the century.[2] In response to these unintended consequences, in 1885, the Women's Temperance Movement was established and dedicated to uplift men to women's sexual standards, i.e. abstinence. A White Ribbon Campaign, in which men who vowed to be pure sported white ribbons on their lapels, was launched.

It was in this social context that Anthony Comstock, (1844-1915), a self-appointed anti-vice crusader from New York, managed to shepherd through Congress a stringent anti-obscenity statute. This statute forbade, among other "impurities," the importing or mailing of contraceptives or contraceptive information. During this period, Comstock-type statutes enacted in many state legislatures forbade the dissemination or, in some cases, even the use of contraceptives. Comstock was so zealous and effective in the enforcement of these laws that by the late 19th century, the subject of contraception had become unmentionable—even in major medical textbooks.

Margaret Sanger (1879-1966), who saw her own mother, age 50, die after 18 pregnancies became a nurse and a leader in the women's right movement. Sanger risked scandal, danger and imprisonment to challenge the legal and cultural obstacles that made controlling fertility difficult and illegal for women here and abroad. Today, adolescents face similar obstacles.

Sanger's first challenges under the Comstock laws focused on health information for adult women. Sanger's view of women in a world ruled by men became the basis for her success. She, too, believed in a woman's duty, but it was "to look the whole world in the face with a go-to-hell look in the eyes, to have an ideal, to speak and act in defiance of convention."

In the fall of 1936, Judge Augustus Hand upheld the overturning of the Comstock prohibition on importing contraceptive devices, opening the federal door for information and making access to contraceptive devices a reality for married women. However, it wouldn't be until the 1965 Supreme Court decision Griswold vs. Connecticut that birth control would be made legal for married couples in every state.

Between 1953 and 1965, the quest for an easy-to-use and effective birth control method was undertaken—not by government-sponsored research, nor even private research typically sponsored by pharmaceutical manufacturers. The social climate supporting such research was still very much rooted in the era of the Comstock laws—socially and morally taboo if not legally taboo. In 1953, research funded by Katherine Dexter McCormick and envisioned by Sanger began on a "pill" that women could take every day to prevent pregnancy. In 1960, the federal Food and Drug Administration approved the first contraceptive pill and many say, launched the sexual revolution.

The '60s not only brought the sexual revolution, but also for the first time, Congress began to understand the importance of family size as a key maternal and child health indicator and a key factor in poverty and economic development. With bipartisan support, Congress passed the first federal law in 1963 to support family planning research. In 1964, Congress established the first grants to support family planning programs under the Office of Economic Opportunity.

These federal victories still ran into problems at the state level. Sometimes, you need to bring in the lawyers. The U.S. Supreme Court's 1965 decision in Griswold vs. Connecticut struck down the last state Comstock law that banned married couples from using contraception. Justice William O. Douglas declared in his opinion, "We deal with a right of privacy older than the Bill of Rights." Unmarried couples were not granted the same right until the U.S. Supreme Court's 1972 decision in Eisenstaat vs. Baird. Again, barriers to family planning services were removed thanks to the judicial system, not the legislative branch.

By 1967, growing bipartisan support in Congress led to the passage of the Title IV-A of the Social Security Act to require state welfare agencies to offer and provide family planning services to women receiving public assistance. By the end of the decade, a sizeable bipartisan consensus had emerged favoring government support of voluntary family planning programs as a means of expanding economic development, alleviating poverty and improving the health of women and their families.

Despite the advances of family planning services, the tragedy of illegal abortion continued to scar the lives of women and their families. Estimates of the annual number of illegal abortions in the 1950s and 1960s range from 200,000 to 1.2 million. Regardless of the number, a few states began repealing abortion bans. In 1967, then-Gov. Ronald Reagan signed The California Therapeutic Abortion Act, legalizing abortion in California.

However, that victory for women's reproductive health did not insure adolescents' equal protection under the law. In 1968, minors were given the right to seek confidential treatment for sexually transmitted diseases and HIV/AIDS. But in 1969, Reagan vetoed a bill allowing teenagers to buy condoms. California was amid a statewide epidemic of gonorrhea, with half of the cases occurring among teenagers. His veto message, "The moral issues inherent in this bill must outweigh whatever medical advantages which might result from its approval" set the stage for morality vs. public health to this day. Fortunately, in 1973, Reagan signed into law legislation allowing minors to seek contraceptive services. Translating reproductive health victories for women into victories for adolescents depends on a variety of factors, but political climate is a key indicator and gives us insight into future controversies.

The '70s era dawned bright for family planning services. Title X of the Public Health Service Act, authored by George Bush Sr., was signed into law by President Nixon, who stated, "No American woman should be denied access to family planning assistance because of her economic condition." In addition to the new federal family planning program, Congress amended Title XIX of the Social Security Act to mandate inclusion of family planning services in all state Medicaid programs. These major public policy advances opened the door for thousands of adolescents and women across the country to have access to comprehensive family planning services. The 1973 U. S. Supreme Court decision, Roe vs. Wade, combined with the family planning expansions, soon gave rise to a conservative backlash.

California's teen birthrates have undergone several distinct periods of change: They declined from the early 1970s to the mid-1970s and changed little from the mid-1970s to the mid-1980s. During that period, California's rate of teen pregnancy was below the national rate. What comes next indicates what happens with a change in political leadership that has authority for programs and services related to reproductive health and especially for adolescent health.

By the 1976 presidential primaries, Reagan expanded his rhetorical range beyond attacks on big government and high taxes to include social issues, thus giving birth to "wedge" politics. Senator Jesse Helms led the assault with the GOP platform statement, and his National Congressional Club PAC raised millions of dollar to bankroll a slate of conservative candidates for Congress. Conservative architect Paul Weyrich reveals his plans, "We are talking about Christianizing America."

The '80s ushered in a conservative movement led by Howard Phillips, Weyrich, Richard Viguerie and Pat Buchanan with a plan to drive moderates out of the Republican Party by issuing "hit lists" of "anti-family" legislators. In 1980, the first religious political scorecard, Christian Voice, scored Congressional candidates on a wide range of issues on which a candidate was expected to take a "pro-moral" stand. The Life Amendment PAC announced a hit list of 18 pro-choice congressional members—most of them Democrats. The result was a Republican tidal wave that resulted in a net gain of 45 congressional seats, 4 governorships and 220 state legislative posts.

The "Christianizing" of America officially began with abstinence-only education leading the religious right agenda. In 1981, the "family values" movement passed the federal Adolescent Family Life Act (AFLA), also known as the "chastity law," which funded educational programs to promote self-discipline and other prudent approaches to adolescent sex. Grant requests for first year funding of $11 million for "chastity education" began pouring into the U.S. Office of Population Affairs from community organizations, including religious institutions. These early grants taught abstinence as the only option for teens. Early grantees often promoted specific religious values prompting a lawsuit filed by the American Civil Liberties Union. Ultimately, an out-of-court settlement in 1993 succeeded in removing the ties to religion as guaranteed by the U.S. Constitution but could do nothing to stop the abstinence-only approach. Current year funding for AFLA is $31 million, and yet there is still no peer-reviewed research that proves it is effective in preventing teen pregnancy.

In 1982, during the last year of his administration, California Gov. Jerry Brown launched a new comprehensive teen pregnancy and parenting program—the Adolescent Family Life Program. Unlike the federal program, the Brown administration recognized the complex social determinants that culminate in teen pregnancy. However, with the election of conservative Gov. George Deukmejian in 1983, family planning services immediately came under direct attack, and services for minors came into focus for conservative organizations. The legacy of the Deukmejian administration after eight years was an overall 8 percent reduction in family planning funding, passage of a parental consent law for minors seeking abortion services (enjoined by a lawsuit from taking effect) and a teen pregnancy rate that increased dramatically from the mid-1980s to the early 1990s. California, like all states, saw a rapid rise in teen pregnancy rates during this period; however, California quickly shot past most states and climbed to 11th highest for teen pregnancy—a dubious distinction that took another decade to reverse. By 2000, California's rates were below the national average, and the state ranked 21st. What policy changes occurred during this time period, and what factors contributed to this change?

In California, the election of Gov. Pete Wilson brought welcome relief for reproductive health advocates. Despite inheriting a massive state deficit and sky-high teen pregnancy rates, Wilson began a systematic, comprehensive approach to teen pregnancy prevention. In addition to the Wilson teen pregnancy prevention initiatives, The California Wellness Foundation (TCWF) launched its own comprehensive Teen Pregnancy Prevention Initiative (TPPI). Uninhibited by the influences of the conservative movement, the TCWF has a unique approach that is not found with any other government-sponsored program. Central to TPPI is the "belief that the problem of teen pregnancy remains largely an adult issue—one that is shaped, determined and perpetuated by the attitudes and behavior of adults and one for which adults bear primary responsibility for solving."

In 1994 in Congress, conservatives, led by California Rep. John Doolittle, introduced an amendment to limit the content of HIV-prevention and sexuality education in school-based programs through a provision in the reauthorization of the Elementary and Secondary Act. Fortunately, the Doolittle attempt ran into technical problems that would have caused four federal statutes to be amended and that ultimately ended his censorship attempt that year.

With a conservative majority in control of both houses of Congress, President Clinton signed into law, "The Personal Responsibility and Work Opportunity Reconciliation Act (PRWORA). The first major reform of the 60-year old federal guarantee of ongoing cash assistance to all qualifying poor families was replaced with time-limited benefits, for which recipients must work, and transferred primary responsibility for the operation of welfare programs to state governments. Conservative critics claimed the former system undermined the "traditional" family by encouraging nonmarital childbearing among poor women. Accordingly, one of the four stated purposes of the new block-grant program was to prevent and reduce the incidence of out-of-wedlock pregnancies. Also included in this reform package were broader social objectives aimed at reforming individuals' sexual behavior and restoring "traditional family norms" not only for those on welfare, but for all Americans.

A cornerstone of PRWORA was another abstinence-only education program. Congressional staff wrote, "The explicit goal of the abstinence-only education programs is to change both behaviors and community standards for the good of the country." American public policy had now come full circle. Just as women leaders in 1870 believed that husbands should practice abstinence as a means of preventing pregnancy, Congress also believes that all individuals, regardless of age, should refrain from sex outside of marriage. To help achieve that goal, Congress guaranteed $50 million annually for grants to states with a requirement that states provide a match of $3 for every $4 of federal funds. This brings public funding to $87 million annually.

Since the passage of the PRWORA, Congress has continued to "invest" in abstinence-only funding through increases to the previous AFL and Special Projects of Regional and National Significance. All grants require states to adhere to a strict eight-point definition of "abstinence education." With the release of President George W. Bush's budget for the next fiscal year, conservative "family values" members have succeeded in their goal of so-called parity between abstinence-only programs and contraceptive services to teens in the Title X program.

What is wrong with this, after all, when everyone agrees that teens should postpone sexual activity? During this period, U.S. teen pregnancy rates have declined nationally and now stand at record low levels. Research suggests that a more realistic "adult" view of adolescent sexuality and more comprehensive approaches to meeting the needs of adolescents as they transition into adulthood has been and continues to be the best way to close the gap in teen pregnancy rates between the United States and other developed countries.

During the '90s, conservative "family values" state policymakers continued a systematic attack on adolescents' access to health education, information and comprehensive health care services. Through control of state legislatures and use of the ballot initiatives, conservative legislators practiced the politics of "incrementalism" and succeeded in winning restrictions on adolescents' access to services. With a few legal victories and defeat of some ballot initiatives, reproductive health advocates were able to stop the most restrictive laws. However, incrementalism remains a successful strategy for conservative "family values" elected officials.

Today, national and public policy research in California are in agreement: Approximately one-quarter of the decline in teen pregnancy rates was due to increased abstinence, and approximately three-quarters of the decline resulted from changes in the behavior of sexually experienced teens. Although research has conclusively demonstrated a comprehensive approach to teen pregnancy prevention, Congress and Bush are still promoting an abstinence-only, family-values agenda that leaves adolescents at risk for unintended pregnancy, sexually transmitted diseases and HIV/AIDS. Conservative legislators playing wedge politics have dealt adolescents a Russian-roulette hand, and it is up to responsible adults to protect adolescents as they transition into adulthood.

Kathy Kneer is president and CEO of Planned Parenthood Affiliates of California (PPAC). Prior to joining Planned Parenthood, Ms. Kneer worked for the March of Dimes Birth Defects Foundation for 18 years, where she advocated on a wide range of maternal and child health policy issues, including expanded access to pregnancy-related health care.

Recent Immigrants and the Role of Parental Involvement in Sexuality Education

By Angel Luis Martinez
International Sex Educator/Trainer

The question put to the roomful of parents, most newcomers to the United States, first elicits a silence that translates as, "Is he serious?" Then come snorts of repressed laughter and finally the shaking of heads. It is November 2003 in San Diego, and the question was a simple one, "How many of you were taught about sex by your parents?" The nonverbal and sublingual responses were not unexpected, nor much different from the responses of similar groups when asked the same question. One or two raised hands indicated affirmative answers, but for most participants, the initial discussion focused on the "ridiculousness" of the question.

Another question: "Who taught your parents about sexual issues?" evokes remarks such as "nobody," and "those things were not talked about."

The fact is the parents of these folks—following the example set for them—did what these parents are doing comprehensive approach to teen pregnancy prevention, Congress and Bush are still promoting an abstinence-only, family-values agenda that leaves adolescents at risk for unintended pregnancy, sexually transmitted diseases and HIV/AIDS. Conservative legislators playing wedge politics have dealt adolescents a Russian-roulette hand, and it is up to responsible adults to protect adolescents as they transition into adulthood.

Kathy Kneer is president and CEO of Planned Parenthood Affiliates of California (PPAC). Prior to joining Planned Parenthood, Ms. Kneer worked for the March of Dimes Birth Defects Foundation for 18 years, where she advocated on a wide range of maternal and child health policy issues, including expanded access to pregnancy-related health care.

Recent Immigrants and the Role of Parental Involvement in Sexuality Education

By Angel Luis Martinez
International Sex Educator/Trainer

The question put to the roomful of parents, most newcomers to the United States, first elicits a silence that translates as, "Is he serious?" Then come snorts of repressed laughter and finally the shaking of heads. It is November 2003 in San Diego, and the question was a simple one, "How many of you were taught about sex by your parents?" The nonverbal and sublingual responses were not unexpected, nor much different from the responses of similar groups when asked the same question. One or two raised hands indicated affirmative answers, but for most participants, the initial discussion focused on the "ridiculousness" of the question.

Another question: "Who taught your parents about sexual issues?" evokes remarks such as "nobody," and "those things were not talked about."

The fact is the parents of these folks—following the example set for them—did what these parents are doing with their children, trying their best. Much like their parents, they are doing what they think is right when it comes to sharing information about sex and hoping that things will turn out all right. They do what they can, but when it comes to sex, sexuality or sexual issues, they react as their parents taught them: That beyond warnings of dire and somewhat obscure consequences, these topics are best avoided. Whether these taboos came from church teachings or cultural proscription, they have been passed down and in important ways shape what many parents do with their children about the dialogue regarding sexuality.

This communication barrier, created in a different age and shaped by the complicity of generations, is in elemental ways reinforced by the nuances and hypocritical sexual messages of our societally approved consumerist sex education.

Consumerist Sex Education

A great many newcomers to the United States come from rural areas, small towns and marginal urban areas. In almost all cases, their defining cultural context included tightly controlled mandates from church regarding sexual conduct as well as cultural norms that reinforced the beliefs that protected family and community values. Once in the United States (often after prodigious efforts), these newcomers find themselves confronting a daunting assortment of challenges that include having to deal with and learn a new language, finding work, finding a place to live and dealing with children confused by drastic change, all while being cut off from support systems of family and community.

Amid all this, they are confronted daily by a barrage of sexual messages that have been concocted for and aimed at a cultural norm that these newcomers are barely beginning to grasp. They become an unprepared segment of the audience for which messages are created and delivered on a massive scale. A significant percentage of these messages are conveyed within subtle and not-so-subtle sexual contexts.

The daily realities of life keep newcomers in work situations where they are either in groups with others like themselves or toiling alone providing services. Social time, what there is of it, calls for taking a breather among those who share language and history. The net effect of this is a practical isolation from the culture whose messages invade their lives and homes in multiple forms—some of which must appear much like science fiction. It is an isolation that inhibits cultural interpretation of the language and sexual images inherent in much of what they experience from the media.

People for whom sexual issues were never discussed in polite company and whose sexual vocabulary is generally circumscribed by elements of off-color humor, double entendres or the passion of swearing—are now coming home to deal with questions they dare not ask. They face concepts that do not fit into their understanding and—most desperately—come home to deal with children who, along with new friends from a confusing array of cultural backgrounds, are being publicly mugged by consumerist sex education. Coming home to children who are surpassing their parents in language acquisition and cultural adaptation, and who are also being influenced by yet another source of sexual content information, institutional sex education.

Institutional Sex Education

A significant number of our schools include, as part of their curriculum, some sort of sexuality education. The quality of this sex education ranges from the abysmal to the "at least up to par with the academic subjects." The inconsistency of the quality of sexuality education is matched only by the ferocity of the conflict that it creates in many communities. Regardless of quality and community acceptance, this institutional aspect of how children learn about sexuality confronts many newcomer families.

One unexpected way in which parents are impacted by this is that schools, often in partnership with social service agencies, confront communities with studies that proclaim parents as the primary educators of their children and either imply or directly command that they play a role. It is a role for which they are wholly unprepared, a role written for a different cast and a role that the dominant culture hasn't done very well with itself.

Consumerist Sex Education vs. Institutional Sex Education

Current federally funded programs support sexuality education that is focused solely on the advocacy of abstinence and preparation for marriage. While young people and their parents are hearing the government-funded abstinence messages on one side, on the other they're being bombarded by the entertainment industry with messages of sexual thoughtlessness, sex without consequences and consumer appetite as means to sexual achievement.

This dichotomy and hypocrisy is not lost upon the newcomer communities. Although they mostly agree with the abstinence until marriage position, they feel lost in terms of dealing with the imagery and messages of media. What can I say, they wonder, that will have a greater impact than a movie or music video? How can I teach respect when the words of the song blaring from the music store command disrespect? How can I honor the purity of relationships when what my kids see and hear tells them that relationships are easily come by, exchanged and disposed of?

In the United States, respect has become just another word—an ineffective concept that has very little currency in a cultural context and is focused on "me first." This concept is guided by governmental and corporate duplicity; however, the word "respect" carries an inestimable value to many newcomers. Respect guides generational conduct, gender behavior and conduct with authority. It is when there is confusion and ambiguity that respect loses power and because there is no substitute for the power it once exerted, what ensues goes far beyond what anyone might call disrespect.

Parental Sex Education

Although they may not have the words, anatomical knowledge or ease of communication, many newcomer parents do participate in the sexual education of their children. There are some clear premises: They want their children to be healthy, protected from abuse, to view sex healthily and they want their children to have a sexual life that is joyful, respectful and loving within a family context. At the same time, they are not unaware of the inherent dangers and barriers. What they lack is the opportunity to learn how to deal with these strange new challenges. They lack the language that their children hear from multiple electronic sources, and they lack the ability to convey what they feel in their hearts and wish to pass on to their children. But this does not deter them from trying; they do what they believe will help their children, even if it means resorting to the faulty admonitions given them by their own parents.

Implication

Social service agencies have begun to allot budget items for the inclusion of parents in a new learning process. However, because of limited resources, these efforts often are entrusted to young people with lots of goodwill and energy but little life experience, training or knowledge, and to semi-prepared community volunteers whose greatest assets complement those that are missing from the younger, hired staff—life experience and the ability to "talk the talk" of their neighbors.

Given the realities and consequences of unprepared for and unprotected sexual activity by young people, and if we truly believe in the importance of the role of parents, then more attention needs to be paid to the "how" of helping parents—especially newcomer parents—learn to decipher the new moralities within which their lives and their children's are lived.

Resources equal to those going to so many "problem centered" programs (that try hard for all of their ineffectiveness), can be allotted to well-thought-out efforts preparing parents. They can help parents understand the vast differences between the world of their adolescence and the one being navigated by their children.

Parents are calling for practical lessons on dealing with difficult questions, help mastering the necessary tools and age-appropriate information. We must not wait until adolescence to intervene. Parents are there from the start and represent the greatest resource to counterbalance the insidious messages of consumerist sex education and the often bureaucratically ambiguous ones of institutional sex education.

All parents will welcome opportunities to enhance their skills, conveying to their children what we once thought love alone could do.

Angel Luis Martinez is an internationally recognized sex educator and trainer. Mr. Martinez has worked with national multisite initiatives, served as technical assistance coordinator to The California Wellness Foundation's Teen Pregnancy Prevention Initiative and trained professionals and others working with young people throughout the United States and Latin America. Mr. Martinez's work includes community organization and development, development of training design and curricula, community health and sexuality/family planning/population issues. He is currently the lead trainer in a multinational project in Latin America to develop and support a new generation of leaders in the field of reproductive health.

Understanding "Abstinence": Implications for Individuals, Programs and Policies

**By Cynthia Dailard,
Senior Public Policy Associate
The Alan Guttmacher Institute**

The word "sex" is commonly acknowledged to mean different things to different people. The same can be said for "abstinence." The varied and potentially conflicting meanings of "abstinence" have significant public health implications now that its promotion has emerged as the current administration's primary answer to pregnancy and sexually transmitted disease (STD) prevention for all people who are not married.

For those willing to probe beneath the surface, critical questions abound. What is abstinence in the first place, and what does it mean to use abstinence as a method of pregnancy or disease prevention? What constitutes abstinence "failure," and can abstinence failure rates be measured comparably to failure rates for other contraceptive methods? What specific behaviors are to be abstained from? And what is known about the effectiveness and potential "side effects" of programs that promote abstinence?

Answering questions about what abstinence means at the individual and programmatic levels and clarifying all of this for policy-makers, remain key challenges. Meeting that challenge should be regarded as a prerequisite for the development of sound and effective programs designed to protect Americans from unintended pregnancy and STDs, including HIV.

Abstinence and Individuals

What does it mean to use abstinence? When used conversationally, most people probably understand abstinence to mean refraining from sexual activity—or, more specifically, vaginal intercourse—for moral or religious reasons. But when it is promoted as a public health strategy to avoid unintended pregnancy or STDs, it takes on a different connotation. Indeed, President Bush has described abstinence as "the surest way, and the only completely effective way, to prevent unwanted pregnancies and sexually transmitted disease." So from a scientific perspective, what does it mean to abstain from sex, and how should the "use" of abstinence as a method of pregnancy or disease prevention be measured?

Population and public health researchers commonly classify people as contraceptive users if they or their partner are consciously using at least one method to avoid unintended pregnancy or STDs. From a scientific standpoint, a person would be an "abstinence user" if he or she intentionally refrained from sexual activity. Thus, the subgroup of people consciously using abstinence as a method of pregnancy or disease prevention is obviously much smaller than the group of people who are not having sex. The size of the population of abstinence users, however, has never been measured, as it has for other methods of contraception.

When does abstinence fail? The definition of an abstinence user also has implications for determining its effectiveness as a method of contraception. The president, in his July 2002 remarks to South Carolina high school students, said: "Let me just be perfectly plain. If you're worried about teenage pregnancy, or if you're worried about sexually transmitted disease, abstinence works every single time." In doing so, he suggested that abstinence is 100 percent effective. But scientifically, is this in fact correct?

Researchers have two different ways of measuring the effectiveness of contraceptive methods. "Perfect use" measures the effectiveness when a contraceptive is used exactly according to clinical guidelines. In contrast, "typical use" measures how effective a method is for the average person who does not always use the method correctly or consistently. For example, women who use oral contraceptives perfectly will experience almost complete protection against pregnancy. However, in the real world, many women find it difficult to take a pill every single day, and pregnancies can and do occur to women who miss one or more pills during a cycle. Thus, although oral contraceptives have a perfect-use effectiveness rate of over 99 percent, their typical-use effectiveness is closer to 92 percent. As a result, eight in 100 women who use oral contraceptives will become pregnant in the first year of use.

When President Bush suggests that abstinence is 100 percent effective, he is implicitly citing its perfect-use rate—and indeed, abstinence is 100 percent effective if "used" with perfect consistency. But common sense suggests that, in the real world, abstinence as a contraceptive method can and does fail. People who intend to remain abstinent may "slip" and have sex unexpectedly. Research is beginning to suggest how difficult abstinence can be to use consistently over time. For example, a recent study presented at the 2003 annual meeting of the American Psychological Society (APS) found that over 60 percent of college students who had pledged virginity during their middle or high school years had broken their vow to remain abstinent until marriage.[1] What is not known is how many of these broken vows represent people consciously choosing to abandon abstinence and initiate sexual activity, and how many are simply typical-use abstinence failures.

To promote abstinence, its proponents frequently cite the allegedly high failure rates of other contraceptive methods, particularly condoms. By contrasting the perfect use of abstinence with the typical use of other contraceptive methods, however, they are comparing apples to oranges. From a public health perspective, it is important both to subject abstinence to the same scientific standards that apply to other contraceptive methods and to make consistent comparisons across methods. However, researchers have never measured the typical-use effectiveness of abstinence. Therefore, it is not known how frequently abstinence fails in the real world or how effective it is compared with other contraceptive methods. This represents a serious knowledge gap. People deserve to have consistent and accurate information about the effectiveness of all contraceptive methods. For example, if they are told that abstinence is 100 percent effective, they should also be told that, if used correctly and consistently, condoms are 97 percent effective in preventing pregnancy. If they are told that condoms fail as much as 14 percent of the time, they should be given a comparable typical-use failure rate for abstinence.

What behaviors should be abstained from? A recent nationally representative survey conducted by the Kaiser Family Foundation and Seventeen magazine found that half of all 15-17 year-olds believed that a person who has oral sex is still a virgin.[2] Even more striking, the APS study found that the majority (55 percent) of college students pledging virginity who said they had kept their vow reported having had oral sex.[3] Although the pledgers generally were somewhat less likely to have had vaginal sex than nonpledgers, they were equally likely to have had oral or anal sex. Because oral sex does not eliminate people's risk of HIV and other STDs, and because anal sex can heighten that risk, being technically abstinent may therefore still leave people vulnerable to disease. Although the media are increasingly reporting that noncoital behaviors are on the rise among young people, no research data exists to confirm this.

Abstinence Education Programs

Defining and communicating what is meant by abstinence are not just academic exercises but are crucial to public health efforts to reduce people's risk of pregnancy and STDs. For example, existing federal and state abstinence-promotion policies typically neglect to define those behaviors to be abstained from. In 2004, the federal government will spend approximately $140 million a year on education programs that exclusively promote "abstinence from sexual activity outside of marriage." The law, however, does not define "sexual activity." As a result, it may have the unintended effect of promoting noncoital behaviors that leave young people at risk. Currently, very little is known about the relationship between abstinence-promotion activities and the prevalence of noncoital activities. This hampers the ability of health professionals and policy-makers to shape effective public health interventions designed to reduce people's risk.

There is no question, however, that increased abstinence—meaning delayed vaginal intercourse among young people—has played a role in reducing teen pregnancy rates in the United States. Research by The Alan Guttmacher Institute (AGI) indicates that 25 percent of the decrease in the U.S. teen pregnancy rate between 1988 and 1995 was due to a decline in the proportion of teenagers who had ever had sex, and 75 percent was due to improved contraceptive use among sexually active teens. Abstinence proponents frequently cite U.S. teen pregnancy declines as "proof" that abstinence-only education programs, which exclude accurate and complete information about contraception, are effective; they argue that these programs should be expanded at home and exported overseas. Yet they say nothing about the effectiveness of programmatic interventions. In fact, significant declines in U.S. teen pregnancy rates occurred prior to the implementation of government-funded programs supporting this particularly restrictive brand of abstinence-only education. Thus, any assumptions about program effectiveness, and the effectiveness of abstinence-only education programs in particular, are misleading and potentially dangerous, but they are nonetheless shaping U.S. policy both here and abroad.

Accordingly, key questions arise about how to measure the success of abstinence-promotion programs. For example, the administration is defining program success for its abstinence-only education grants to community and faith-based organizations in terms of shaping young people's intentions and attitudes with regard to future sexual activity. In contrast, most public health experts stress the importance of achieving desired behavioral outcomes such as delayed sexual activity.

To date, however, no education program in this country focusing exclusively on abstinence has shown success in delaying sexual activity. Perhaps some will in the future. In the meantime, considerable scientific evidence already demonstrates that certain types of programs that include information about both abstinence and contraception help teens delay sexual activity, have fewer sexual partners and increase contraceptive use when they begin having sex. It is not clear what it is about these programs that leads teens to delay—a question that researchers need to explore. What is clear, however, is that no program of any kind has ever shown success in convincing young people to postpone sex from age 17, when they typically first have intercourse, until marriage, which typically occurs at age 25 for women and

27 for men. Nor is there any evidence that the "wait until marriage" message has any impact on young people's decisions regarding sexual activity. This suggests that scarce public dollars could be better spent on programs that have been proven to achieve delays in sexual activity of any duration, rather than on programs that stress abstinence until marriage.

Finally, there is the question of whether delays in sexual activity might come at an unacceptable price. This is raised by research indicating that although some teens promising to abstain from sex until marriage delayed sexual activity by an average of 18 months, they were more likely to have unprotected sex when they broke their pledge than those who never pledged virginity in the first place. Thus, might strategies to promote abstinence inadvertently heighten the risks for people when they eventually become sexually active?

Difficult as it may be, answering these key questions regarding abstinence eventually will be necessary for the development of sound and effective programs and policies. At a minimum, the existing lack of common understanding hampers the ability of the public and policy makers to fully assess whether abstinence and abstinence education are viable and realistic public health and public policy approaches to reducing unintended pregnancies and HIV/STDs.

Reproduced with the permission of The Alan Guttmacher Institute from: Dailard C., Understanding abstinence: Implications for Individuals, Programs and Policies, The Guttmacher Report on Public Policy, 6(5): 4-6, 2003.

Cynthia Dailard is senior public policy associate at The Alan Guttmacher Institute's Washington, D.C., office and is responsible for issues related to domestic family planning programs, sexuality education and insurance coverage of contraception. Ms. Dailard previously served as associate director for domestic policy in the Clinton

White House, legislative assistant and counsel to United State Senator Olympia Snowe (R-ME), and staff attorney at the National Women's Law Center.

Reclaiming Abstinence Education

By Tom Klaus, Founder/President
Legacy Resource Group

Abstinence education is an important aspect of comprehensive sexuality education. Can it be stated any more plainly than that? Any questions about what it means? OK, for you in the back row: *Even the most vocal proponents of comprehensive sexuality education (CSE) understand and appreciate the need to promote sexual abstinence.*

In its "Adolescence and Abstinence Fact Sheet" the Sexuality Information and Education Council of the United States (SIECUS) clearly states, "Adolescents should be encouraged to delay sexual behaviors until they are physically, cognitively and emotionally ready for mature sexual relationships and their consequences." SIECUS is the organization that wrote the guidelines for CSE, which has helped form similar statements at the state and local level. Advocates For Youth, the driving force behind the "Rights, Respect and Responsibility Campaign" even offers a lesson plan for promoting abstinence titled "Teaching Abstinence as a Part of Comprehensive Sexuality Education: What Is Abstinence?" Question: If those of us who support CSE have been so pro-abstinence, why has the issue gotten away from us and landed in the hands of the abstinence-only and abstinence-until-marriage crowd?

I may not have a definitive answer, but I do have a definitive opinion. While we were busy defending Comprehensive Sexuality Education, we let others claim abstinence, redefine it outside the context of CSE and promote it as something separate, if not actually in opposition to, CSE. In short, we gave it away. To reclaim it—and I feel strongly that we should—we must act now because abstinence is on the move again. This time it is moving not just from us, but from the abs-only/abs-until-marriage folks, too.

And whom is it moving to? Youth and adolescents. But why should that concern us? After all, we believe in the ability of youth to make wise and appropriate decisions, although we usually add a disclaimer along the lines of "when they have complete and accurate information." Ownership of abstinence is a concern now because it is being defined in some circles in such a way that it may actually become a risky sexual behavior. This is happening because youth and adolescents are not getting complete, accurate information. They also are discouraged by the "abstinence-only until marriage" message because it seems such a long way off.

Results from a recent study conducted in the heartland of America, smack dab on the buckle of the Bible belt, may offer some support for this idea. Northern Kentucky University researcher and psychologist Angela Lipsitz reported that her study of 600 teens indicated:

- Over half of the teens believed a person should still be considered abstinent after engaging in oral sex;
- 61 percent of those who had taken abstinence or virginity pledges broke them within a year;
- Over half of the 39 percent who did not "break" their pledges engaged in oral sex.

Dr. Lipsitz is not alone in her findings. Both anecdotal and research evidence from around the United States concur that abstinence once again is being claimed and redefined—this time by youth and adolescents—and redefined in a way that allows for other intimate sexual behaviors that can be dangerous if practiced without protection.

Clearly, for the sake of youth and adolescents, we must reclaim the abstinence message in a way that is consistent with a commitment to Comprehensive Sexuality Education.

First, we must take the initiative in clearly defining sexual intimacy and sexual abstinence in a way that adolescents can understand. Both sexual intimacy and sexual abstinence must be defined because to understand one requires understanding the other. This may not be a comfortable fact for adults to embrace, but it is true. You can't effectively teach about one without teaching about the other.

This may sound like a reasonable idea, but a start is needed. I offer a starting place for both definitions. Although not perfect, they allow us to cross a frontier where the public health education community has been reluctant to venture.

Sexual Intimacy: Sexual intimacy is any sexually physical interaction, in which bodily fluids can be exchanged, that occurs between two or more people that may include, but is not limited to:

- Sexual intercourse—inserting penis into vagina;
- Anal sex—inserting penis into anus;
- Oral sex—stimulating the penis, vagina or clitoris using another's mouth or tongue;
- Penetration—inserting digits (fingers and toes) or objects into vagina or anus;
- Skin to skin touching in such a way that allows seminal fluid, vaginal secretions, or secretion from open sores to be exchanged from one person to another.

Sexual Abstinence: Sexual abstinence is the conscious choice made by partners to hold off, postpone or delay engaging in sexual intimacy for the purpose(s) of supporting one's:

- Health—avoiding unplanned pregnancy or sexually transmitted infections/diseases;
- Aspirations—attaining specific academic, social or personal goals free of the commitment required to establish and maintain a healthy intimate sexual relationship;
- Values—being consistent with one's personal, moral, ethical or faith convictions.

Affirming the definitions is less important than motivating people to tackle the issue. All of us—whether we support CSE or abstinence-only approaches—must get real about the need for clear definitions that youth and adolescents can use to set their own boundaries.

Second, let's address sexual abstinence as another contraceptive technology. Regardless of how we view sexual abstinence philosophically, there should be no disagreement that it will work effectively only under three conditions.

1. *Consistent usage:* You can't be abstinent on Monday, Wednesday and Friday but not on Tuesday, Thursday or Saturday and expect it to work. The commitment to sexual abstinence is the same commitment a couple makes to the use of other contraceptive technologies—birth control pill, condom, diaphragm, etc. It must be used every day, or every time sex is a possibility.
2. *Correct usage*: Every contraceptive technology has clear instructions—except sexual abstinence. Telling youth and adolescents to "wait until marriage" or to "wait until you are more mature and know about the responsibilities" are not effective strategies. Both misunderstand the basics of

adolescent development. Marriage seems a long time off to an adolescent whose concept of time is distorted by a longing to become an adult, and besides, telling youth and adolescents when it is okay to engage in sexual intimacy is not the same as giving them instructions. This leads back to the first point, that we must start giving them instructions by providing clear definitions.
3. *Joint usage:* Sexual abstinence doesn't usually work when only one person in the partnership chooses it. Optimally, both have to be committed to its consistent and correct usage. Ideally, the commitment level will be near equal so the relationship can grow and develop in a way that will, in due time, support a healthy sexual intimacy.

If we begin thinking of sexual abstinence as contraceptive technology, we also must think realistically about its success and failure rates. "Sexual abstinence is the only thing that is 100 percent effective in preventing unplanned teen pregnancy and STDs" sounds good, but it is untrue. It is just as accurate to say "Death is 100 percent effective in preventing unplanned teen pregnancy and STDs" but it certainly doesn't sound good. Just because something makes a good sound bite doesn't make it a good strategy.

We must get real about the effectiveness of sexual abstinence. Is it 100 percent effective? Yes, but only when the partners use it correctly and consistently. In fact, there is little research to tell us the success or failure rate of sexual abstinence in actual practice. A 1999 article published in Family Planning Perspectives[1] by Fu, Darroch, Haas and Ranjit indicates that periodic abstinence (a form of abstinence but not as defined above) failed more often than condoms, implants, injections or birth control pills. In a 12 month period, 26.3 percent of unmarried, not cohabitating women under age 20 experienced contraceptive failure using periodic abstinence versus 1.4 percent of implant users, 2.4 percent of injectable users, 7.6 percent of birth control pill users and 14 percent of condom users. Only withdrawal (26.4 percent) and spermicides (29.4 percent) did worse than periodic abstinence.

In addition, Haignere, Gold and McDaniel in "Adolescent Use of Condoms and Abstinence: Are We Sure We Are Teaching What is Safe?"[2] remind us that contraceptive technologies have two kinds of failure rates—user-failure and method-failure. The method-failure rate of latex condoms is very, very low because of the low number of defects (despite the myth of microscopic holes in latex condoms). However, the user-failure rate is significantly higher because condoms may not be used correctly. If we consider sexual abstinence in the same light, we'd have to agree that it has a zero percent method-failure rate. But if the user-failure rate for sexual abstinence is based on the percentage of people who intend (or pledge) to practice sexual abstinence but don't, the failure-rate for sexual abstinence may be very high. As Lipsitz's study suggests, it may be as high as 61 percent within the first 12 months of the pledge.

All things considered, a strong case still can be made for treating sexual abstinence as a contraceptive technology worthy of praise for its effectiveness, with the qualifying caution that partners must use it correctly and consistently.

Third point—let's reclaim abstinence education by committing to doing it better than anyone else. One can argue what "better" means, and it can be argued that those committed to CSE should be able to teach sexual abstinence better than anyone else. After all, we have the experience, the research and the knowledge. But it takes two other factors that I'm not sure we have.

Truth. Truth can be a scary word. It conjures up images of people who are loud, arrogant, rigid and downright unpleasant to be near. However, there is also a different image, the image of a person who takes the stand in a trial and is sworn to "tell the truth, the whole truth and nothing but the truth." When we stand before children, youth and adolescents to teach about sexual abstinence, we should be driven by the same oath.

- *Tell the truth:* The worst thing we can do is lie to kids. Although most of us never would intentionally, we might pay "lip-service" to sexual abstinence because we think it is "politically correct" or our funding is dependent upon it. But adolescents know it when adults play games. If we don't have our heart in it, they'll know, and it will come across as a lie. We can put our hearts into it, once we reclaim abstinence education as the important part of CSE we know it is.
- *Tell the Whole Truth:* To tell the whole truth is to give youth and adolescents all the information they need, not just the information you are comfortable delivering or what other even less-comfortable adults think kids should have. Correct information about sexual intimacy is essential to practicing sexual abstinence consistently.
- *Tell Nothing But The Truth:* We don't like seeing fear-based approaches being used with youth and adolescents in any sexuality education but especially in abstinence education. We all have stories to tell of abstinence educators who used fear and shame-based techniques to get kids to sign abstinence pledges and scare parents into "talking" (read "lecture") to their kids about the dangers of sex—protected or unprotected. Because we may cringe at this, our own presentations may be skewed because we don't want to do this to kids. This may result in an unintentional distortion of the truth of our own. We may fail to give due weight to the dangers of sex that are real. To tell nothing but the truth is to be honest and balanced in our messages on both the benefits and dangers of sex.

Will. We won't reclaim abstinence education unless we find the will to do so. This will not be easy, and it may take time, but much is at stake. My youngest son went off to college this fall, leaving behind his dog, his home and his first love. He has been glad to be away from home, but he has missed his dog and pines for his love. The distance between school and home has brought us closer together via the telephone. We talk at least once a week and for surprising periods of time—often 45 minutes to an hour. We talk about everything, including sex.

As a school-age boy, my son traveled with me when I spoke to youth groups or trained and taught other sexuality educators. He heard nearly all of my presentations, even to the point where he might have actually been able to repeat one or two from memory. Before he went off to college, the only other time we directly talked about sex was when he was entering high school. He had said to me, "Dad, I've decided what I want for myself about sex. I want to be abstinent until I get married." Then he paused, looked square into my eyes and said, "But, dad, if I change my mind, I know how to use a condom, and I will."

I haven't figured out if he is changing his mind, now that he is in college, but I do know that he is thinking carefully about that earlier decision. He is, even at the age of 19, a deeply spiritual man who tries to weigh life decisions by the ethic he espouses. Recently, he told me: "Even if I decided it was OK for me to have sex before I get married, I know I couldn't just have sex just to have sex. It would have to be with someone I care about and who cares about me. It has to mean something."

A few years ago, I decided I would reclaim the abstinence message—at least for my own son. At the time, I wasn't sure if it would be effective. It was tempting to let him get just the "abstinence-only-until-marriage" message from his public school and his faith community, even though I was unsatisfied with both the methodology and content. It would have been easier, but it didn't seem responsible as a parent.

The children, youth and adolescents we work with may not be our own children. Our days are so full that it usually will seem easier to just let others shape the abstinence message. As public servants, social workers, counselors, teachers, youth workers, child advocates and policy-makers, we still have to get real with ourselves about our responsibility. Not just for our own kids but also for all kids, it is time for us to reclaim abstinence education.

Tom Klaus is founder and president of Legacy Resource Group, which provides training, program resources and consultation to communities and youth-serving groups nationwide. Mr. Klaus has been involved in professional youth work as a consultant, speaker, minister, program developer and administrator for more than 25 years.

Healthy Adolescent Sexuality

By Tamara Kreinin, M.H.S.A., President/CEO
Sexuality Information and
Education Council of the United States

Successful strategies for teenage pregnancy prevention in the United States have eluded us for decades. Identified repeatedly as a key factor in our high rates of child poverty and a critical social issue, teen pregnancy prevention largely has received lip service from our elected officials. The dollars invested in prevention are minimal compared with the high costs that are associated with adolescent pregnancy. Despite many programmatic efforts, the United States continues to have the highest rates of teenage pregnancy of any industrialized nation.

We have experienced declines in teen pregnancy and birthrates over the past 10 years, yet we cannot become complacent. Every year, a new generation of teens will face the challenges of navigating relationships and making decisions about sexuality. These young people will experience new developmental stages and pressures from the external environment, such as their peers and the media, at many points during their teen years. Some of the speculated reasons for the declines in teen pregnancy and birthrates, such as HIV/AIDS prevention and advocacy and a strong economy, are shifting.

Young people are not as aware as they once were of the devastation caused by HIV/AIDS and thus may not be as cautious in their sexual behaviors. Many of the HIV/AIDS-prevention programs that may have contributed to decreasing rates of teen pregnancy are under attack from conservative political action groups and elected officials. Nearly $1 billion has been spent by federal and state government(s) for abstinence-only-until-marriage programs, (many of which send false messages to teens, including that condoms do not work) rather than programs that have been evaluated as effective. We don't yet know the impact this will have. We also are seeing increases in pregnancy rates among select teen populations such as Latina girls (this could have a significant impact long term because young Latino/a youth are a demographic that continues to increase).

We have identified some promising programs and in a few instances replicated them. However, more often than not, programs receive praise and positive evaluations and then are not given their due because they are considered "too expensive or too controversial." We as a nation have not taken the stance that teenage pregnancy is unacceptable other than to "wag our finger" at the teens themselves. Thus, adults frequently do not support teens in such a way that they delay pregnancy. We have not created a social norm that communicates to our young people consistently that we have other things for them to do than get pregnant. Nor have we set a standard for what we want for our youth. In this vacuum, the media have stepped in and increasingly sexualized younger and younger children. At the same time, we are denying them accurate information and an opportunity to discuss and process what they see and experience around them. This combination sets up our young people for victimization and confusion.

There is no "magic bullet" for prevention of unplanned

pregnancy. Teenage pregnancy and teenage sexuality are complicated and can be successfully addressed only with an array of strategies. Further, we must look at the root causes of teenage pregnancy such as poverty and a poor educational system. We must not ignore the complexity of teens' lives. There is much to be learned from research, the few well-evaluated, effective programs and by listening to our young people.

I contend that we must change the conversation. We spend far too much time berating our youth for their behaviors and discussing the problems we want to stop. Rather, we should begin to reach beyond simply avoiding a pregnancy (or disease for that matter) and ask what we want for our young people and how we as adults can help get them there. I submit that we want them to have the support such that they grow up to be productive members of society and have a healthy view of sexuality, their own and others'. Thus, in thinking about creative solutions we must explore first what a sexually health adolescent looks like and next how we as adults, communities and society can best support our young people so that they achieve these outcomes.

We want our young people to understand the consequences of sexual activity. However, we also want them to have a positive view of sexuality, whether they are sexually active as teens or they delay sexual activity until they are in a committed relationship or married.

What does a sexually healthy adolescent look like?

A sexually healthy adolescent has a positive view of his/her sexuality. This goes well beyond avoiding pregnancy and disease. S/he has the tools and motivation to avoid both and also appreciates that sexuality is a natural and healthy part of life. There are several elements to the definition of a sexually healthy adolescent, which include having information and skills

and reflecting one's values and attitudes—this will change based on age and stage of development.

The following provides a starting point.

A sexually healthy adolescent:

Is well-informed about a broad range of sexual health topics

All teens should have medically accurate information about a variety of sexual health topics at age and developmentally appropriate intervals. This includes an understanding of anatomy and reproduction, an understanding of the process of puberty, an awareness of the changes their own bodies will undergo, the knowledge that these changes are normal, the facts about reproduction, the facts about sexually transmitted diseases and all aspects of disease and pregnancy prevention, physiology including sexual responses and sexual behavior. They understand that sexuality is a natural and healthy part of their growth and development throughout life.

Knows when and where to seek additional information and health care

Young people need to know and feel that no question is a bad question and that at any point in time they can ask for more information. Not only should they have trusted adults to seek out for information, they should know that if the adults don't have the answers, the adults will find out and get back to them or lead them to accurate resources. Further, they need to know where else they can get information (such as the library, Internet, health clinics) and how to evaluate sources of information.

Teens also need to know how to access medical care. Ideally their health care visits will be preventative in nature, but they also must know that if they suspect that they have a disease or are pregnant, it is important to seek testing and treatment early and that many diseases can be treated and are curable. The sexually healthy teen also knows that s/he has the right to a health care provider that makes him/her comfortable and can change providers if this is not the case. They know their legal rights to health care and who the providers are in their area.

Understands gender roles

As they develop, teens increasingly will understand gender-related issues and forge their own identity and sense of self. They will have the ability to assess the various and conflicting roles that society often assigns based on gender and make appropriate choices within the context of their values and culture. They know that these choices can change over time. They interact and communicate with each gender comfortably and respectfully. They believe that regardless of gender, everyone has equal rights and responsibilities in relationships (sexual and nonsexual). They treat their peers with respect regardless of their choices.

Understands sexual orientation and identity

They begin to assess their own orientation and also understand, accept and respect other people's sexual orientation. They understand how and why people are gay/lesbian/bisexual/transgender, myths about sexual orientation, different values and where to go for support. They also understand that sexual orientation can be confusing and know how to get support to help sort out their feelings and values.

Has a positive body image and sense of self

They take pride in and have an appreciation of their own body. They understand that bodies grow and change during puberty. They understand that all bodies are different, all bodies are special including those that are disabled and that each person can be proud of his/her own special qualities. They also know that the size and shape of a penis or breasts does not affect reproductive ability or the ability to be a good sexual partner. They understand that the media portrays people with images that most people do not fit, and they do not have the expectation of fitting these images. They realize that their value and the value of others are not based on appearance.

Can assess values and attitudes related to sexuality

They know their own values and views about sexuality and have the ability to reflect on the views and values of their family, religion, culture and community and integrate them into their own views. They feel empowered to act on those views.

They understand outside pressures from various influences, such as the media, peers, family, religion and culture. They can distinguish how their own values and desires are similar and different and feel able to follow their own path.

Has the skills to negotiate relationships

This teen has the opportunity to learn and practice skills, including decision-making, critical thinking, refusal and negotiation and communication skills. Teens not only understand these skills, they have the opportunity to discuss and practice them. They feel empowered to use these skills.

Understands his/her rights in a sexual relationship

They understand their rights related to sexual and reproductive health, including the right to information and services; the right to set boundaries about sexual activity; the right to have those boundaries respected; the right to noncoercive, nonviolent, consensual, honest and mutually pleasurable sexual activity. They have the right to be protected from pregnancy and/or disease as relevant to the sexual behavior. They have the ability to express affection and love at their own comfort level. They have the understanding that the reason to be sexual is pleasure and intimacy.

Understands the potential consequences of sexual activity

They understand that sexual activity has positive and negative consequences that are both physical and emotional. They understand that it is important to be physically and emotionally prepared to be sexually active and to be able to discuss decisions about sexual activity with their partner. They also are aware that drug and alcohol use can impair decision-making. They feel empowered to say and act on what they do and do not want. And they know that they can change their mind at any point. They also know how to seek help if they feel like they have experienced negative consequences such as rape or abuse.

They understand the potential impact of outside influences (such as the media and peers) on sexual behaviors and are able to differentiate their own values and desires from these influences.

Fundamentally, all of these aspects of a sexually healthy adolescent are related to having access to information and services, being able to assess one's values and attitudes and feeling empowered. It is our responsibility as a society and as adults to create an environment in which adolescents can be sexually healthy.

How Can Adults Foster Sexually Healthy Adolescents?

Adults have a responsibility to help young people understand and accept their sexuality as they grow up. It is unfair to expect adolescents to come upon these skills by themselves. Thus, to help foster sexually healthy adolescents, adults must play an active role. Adults must assure that teens have access to accurate information and services, the opportunity to discuss attitudes and values, the opportunity to learn and practice skills, ongoing support and guidance and positive role models.

Parents and caregivers can have open communication with their children

Parents and caregivers first should identify their own values and decide how they are going to approach sexuality with their children, then start at an early age making the topic comfortable and being easily accessible in discussing these issues. Parents/caregivers should talk early and often about not only the basics of anatomy, physiology and reproduction, but also about relationships, dating and attitudes and values about sexuality. They also should help their children reflect on the influences they will encounter in day-to-day life (such as media and peers). If a parent/caregiver is so uncomfortable with these topics or feels their adolescent really is not open to discussion, then they should identify other adults and resources in the teen's life to help with these conversations. Parents' own relationships and behaviors also serve as critical role models

Schools can provide high quality comprehensive sexuality education

Children and youth need age-appropriate comprehensive sexuality education. This should assist children in having a positive view of sexuality, provide them with information and skills related to their sexual health and help them make decisions and negotiate relationships. Effective comprehensive sexuality education must be taught by well-trained teachers who are comfortable with the material and with all students. It must be taught in multiple sessions and through a variety of media, be experiential, skill-based and culturally sensitive and be relevant to all youth, regardless of culture and sexual orientation. It must discuss social influences and pressures and address controversial issues.

Faith communities can address sexuality-related issues

Faith communities provide a great opportunity for education and discussion of values. Many denominations have developed curricula. They can incorporate sexuality education into their programming for children and youth. They also can offer programs to help and support parents and caregivers in conversations with their children. Further, faith communities can offer programming to help young people develop a strong sense of self and their futures.

Community programs can provide information and services

Community programs can offer high quality youth development programs to help young people develop the motivation and skills to envision productive futures and also to become sexually healthy. Youth development programs can infuse their programming with sexuality education. Staff can be trained to integrate sexuality information and referrals throughout youth development programs. These programs must be accessible to all young people, safe and inviting.

Health care services can be accessible and available

Communities must provide primary health care, reproductive health care and mental health services that are accessible for all adolescents. These services can be school-based or linked and also must be accessible to teens who are not in school. The hours and location must be convenient and the space and staff inviting to all teens. Services must be affordable and confidential. Young people should be involved in designing the programs and providing ongoing feedback.

Young people are listened to and respected

Adults must listen to young people and respect their perspective and points of view. They must create forums, both formal and informal, for listening to youth and understanding the context of their lives including current youth culture in their community. They must demonstrate that they value, respect, accept and trust young people and try to understand an adolescent's point of view even if it differs from their own.

Stigma and discrimination are countered

At all levels from home to community institutions, we must work to counter stigma and discrimination. For young people, the adults must actively model acceptance and respect for all.

Culture, tradition and experience is considered in programming

With increasing immigration and migration, cultural context is critical. Programs must understand, consider and incorporate history, traditions and culture of all participants. We must respect diversity and empower and educate young people within the context of their own culture, tradition and experience while also acknowledging that they reside in the United States.

What Questions Must We Pose to Help Foster Sexually Healthy Adolescents?

- Do we understand and pay attention to the particular culture of and influences on the teens in our community?

- Do our young people have a voice?
- Are we addressing our programs and policies both to young women and men?
- Are we attending to the particular needs of both young women and men?
- Are our children and youth receiving high quality age-appropriate comprehensive sexuality education in school and in other appropriate venues?
- Are parents and caregivers in an ongoing conversation with their youth?
- Are we as a community supporting parents in their role as sexuality educators?
- Are reproductive services available and accessible to young women and men in the community?
- Do our young people have the support to succeed in school?
- Do our young people have enough to do outside school?

If we truly are to solve this problem, we must combat complacency. We must not allow conflict to impede action; we must develop a plan and stay focused. We must create political will not only to prevent teen pregnancy, but also to attain positive outcomes for our young people. We must listen to our young people carefully. Finally, we as adults must remember, teen pregnancy is also an adult problem, and we must be leaders in finding the solutions.

Tamara Kreinin, M.H.S.A. is president and CEO of the Sexuality Information and Education Council of the United States. Ms. Kreinin has more than 20 years of experience in health care and human services, including serving as director of state and local affairs at The National Campaign to Prevent Teen Pregnancy and senior program associate at the Southern Regional Project on Infant Mortality.

A Matter of Faith: Reaching Out to Faith Communities for Teenage Pregnancy Prevention

**By the Rev. Debra W. Haffner, MPH, M.Div., Director
Religious Institute on Sexual Morality, Justice, and Healing**

After nearly 20 years as a sexuality educator and expert in adolescent sexuality, I began to study for the ministry. In May 2003, after nearly seven years of intense preparation, I was ordained as a Unitarian Universalist minister. People are often surprised to find out that I identify myself as a sexologist and a minister, believing that the combination is an oxymoron. But my call to ministry grows out of my belief that our spirituality is one of God's most life-fulfilling and life-giving gifts and that our sexuality and spirituality are inexorably linked.

Many of us in the reproductive health field are wary of organized religion. We have been bruised in our struggles with the religious right in battles about abortion, sexuality education, sexual orientation and contraception. Or perhaps we have had personal experiences with organized religion that have alienated us. Others of us have had experiences that support reaching out to religious leaders and communities of faith, recognizing that the religious right does not represent the majority of faith traditions committed to young people's sexual and reproductive health needs. In this chapter, I offer a rationale for involving faith communities in teenage pregnancy prevention and suggestions both to the faith community on serving young people's sexual health needs and to adolescent pregnancy prevention service providers for reaching out to faith communities.

Rationale

With the exception of the public schools, faith-based institutions serve more young people than any other community setting. More than 60 percent of American teens report that they spend at least one hour per week in activities in a church or synagogue, and three-quarters of teens say religion is at least somewhat important to them, including almost half who say it is very important.[1]

Participation in a religious setting actually may protect young people against premature involvement in sexual behaviors. In a review of more than 50 studies of the impact of religion on sexual behavior, Dr. Brian Wilcox and colleagues concluded that "more frequent religious attendance is associated with later initiation of sexual intercourse for white males and for females across racial/ethnic groups [and] more conservative sexual attitudes and a decreased frequency of sexual intercourse."[2] Sexually active African American teenage girls who attend church frequently, pray and partake in other religious activities are less likely to engage in sexually risky behaviors than their less-religious peers. Religious teen females were 50 percent more likely to wait to have intercourse and 80 percent more likely to use a condom the last time they had sex than their less-religious peers.[3] Teens are twice as likely to cite their "morals, values and religious beliefs" as affecting their decision about whether to have intercourse than any other single factor.[4] In a study of more than 600 congregations, youth from congregations that include information about contraception as part of the religious education curriculum report virtually no instances of pregnancy.[5]

Religious youth who did not engage in adolescent sexual intercourse shared characteristics beyond their simple involvement in a religious institution. According to a statistical analysis of more than 6000 young people who participate in religious institutions, those who are least likely to have intercourse:

- Attend religious services one or more times a week,
- Pray daily,
- Are engaged in at least one other congregational activity besides worship;
- Say that the teachings of the congregation and/or Scripture have a lot of influence on their sexual decision-making and that they learned these teachings from the congregation;
- Feel a strong connection with congregational leaders and other youth in the congregation;
- Feel that adults who work with them portray sexuality in a healthy and positive manner;
- Say their congregation encourages abstinence from intercourse for high-school-age teens.[6]

Unfortunately, most studies also indicate that religious youth are less likely to use contraception.[7] And sexually abstinent youth are reporting high levels of involvement in noncoital behaviors. In one study, nearly one-third of the virgins had had oral sex, half had been nude with a person of the other gender, and almost three-quarters had participated in genital fondling.[8]

Disappointingly, but perhaps not surprisingly, only 6 percent of teens say that ministers, rabbis or other religious leaders influence their decisions about sex.[9] Only 14 percent of clergy say that their congregation offers a reasonably comprehensive approach to sexuality education, and 37 percent say the congregation does almost nothing. Fewer than one in six religious youths say that their faith-based institution offers them significant information on birth control, STD prevention, HIV prevention, rape or homosexuality.[10]

Teens and clergy disagree about the sexuality education that is being offered. Although 73 percent of clergy said that their congregation portrays sexuality in a positive and healthy way, only 46 percent of the teens in those same congregations agreed. Although clergy and religious advisers rate their sexuality education programs as fair to good, youth in these programs rate them as poor.[11]

Faith Communities and Sexuality Education

The good news is that three-quarters of adults and teens believe that churches and other faith communities should do more to help prevent teen pregnancy.[12] Many denominations have made a commitment to sexuality education for young people. Several have passed policies that encourage their congregations to include sexuality education in the religious education program. These include American Baptist Churches in the U.S.A., the Central Conference of American Rabbis, the Christian Church (Disciples of Christ), the Episcopal Church, the Mennonite Church, the Presbyterian Church (U.S.A.), the Unitarian Universalist Association, the United Church of Christ, the United Methodist Church and the United Synagogue of Conservative Judaism.[13]

Indeed, more than 30 years ago, the National Council of Churches' Commission on Marriage and Family, the

Synagogue Council of America's Committee on Family and the United States Catholic Conference called upon churches and synagogues to become actively involved in sexuality education within their congregations and their communities.

Many denominations have produced sexuality education curricula; the majority are aimed at adolescents. Many easily could be adapted for other faith communities. There are also national organizations that have produced curricula for use in an interfaith setting. (An annotated list of curricula for adolescents developed for use in faith communities can be found at *www.religiousinstitute.org*). The Unitarian Universalist Association and the United Church of Christ collaborated on a life-span sexuality education program, which begins in kindergarten and includes age-appropriate curricula through adulthood, which is based on the Guidelines for Comprehensive Sexuality Education.

Sexuality education programs in religious institutions have a unique opportunity to teach values within the theological commitments of the denomination. Although each congregation or denomination, depending on polity, will seek to develop a curriculum consistent with its own tradition, certain values transcend denominational frameworks. A colloquium of theologians convened by the Religious Institute on Sexual Morality, Justice and Healing identified that any sexuality education program should:

- Emphasize responsibility, rights, ethics and justice;
- Affirm the dignity and worth of all persons;
- Teach that sexuality includes physical, ethical, social, psychological, emotional and spiritual dimensions;
- Complement the education provided by parents and faith communities—parents should be asked to give written permission before a program begins, and homework assignments can encourage parent/child communication;

- Explicitly identify the values that underline the program;
- Teach that decisions about sexual behaviors should be based on moral and ethical values, as well as considerations of physical and emotional health;
- Affirm the goodness of sexuality while acknowledging its risks and dangers;
- Introduce with respect the differing sides of controversial sexual issues.[14]

Many congregations and denominations may not be ready to adopt a comprehensive sexuality education program, kindergarten through high school. Still, there are less-intensive activities that a congregation can offer to support the sexual health and development of youth. These may include:

- Using an outside consultant periodically from the health department, local AIDS organization or local Planned Parenthood to speak with youth groups about sexuality issues;
- Facilitating youth group members' participation in community activities that relate to sexuality issues—for example, young people can volunteer at a family planning clinic, AIDS organization, children's hospital, adoption agency or hotline for young people;
- Providing support groups for young people, including groups for those whose parents are going through divorce, dealing with sexual orientation, eating disorder and body-image issues; leaders of "drop in" programs should have experience and training to handle teen sexuality issues;
- Including pamphlets about sexual health services in youth center spaces and hanging posters for young people from such organizations as the National AIDS Clearinghouse, the National Campaign To Prevent

Teenage Pregnancy and PFLAG (Parents and Friends of Lesbians and Gays);
- Training members of high school youth groups to provide education about peer pressure on dating, drugs, drinking and sex to middle school students and pre-adolescents—modeling safe behaviors will benefit both groups;
- Having movie nights with such themes as relationships, coming-of-age stories, marriage, friendships and sexual orientation—these can be intergenerational evenings that include discussion between youth and adults after the movie;
- Providing small group sessions or worship services for high school and middle school youth that focus on such issues as body image, peer pressure, relationships with parents and friendships—young people should be given opportunities to talk among themselves and with trained leaders about the pressures they face;
- Providing a Bible study group for teens that focuses on texts with sexual themes and issues;
- Offering programs for parents and middle school students on adjusting to the challenges of puberty and adolescence, as well as maintaining open lines of communication through the teen years;
- Working with youth ministers and religious educators from other congregations to develop community programming;
- Opening youth programming to young people in the surrounding community.[15]

Outreach to Faith Communities

Community-based teenage pregnancy prevention organizations also can reach out to faith communities to involve them in their work. Some possible activities include:

1) Becoming active in one's own faith community on sexuality issues. Offer to work with the lay and religious leaders on helping them become sexually healthy faith communities. (The Religious Institute publishes a monograph, "A Time To Build: Creating Sexually Healthy Faith Communities" that may be helpful.) Volunteer to do youth education and adult education programs on sexuality issues. Establish a committee to develop policies to assure that yours is a safe congregation or a welcoming congregation. Live your faith by offering your sexology.
2) Identify supportive clergy and supportive congregations in your community. Invite clergy to be on your advisory boards. Make sure you have referral sources to rabbis, ministers and priests, who are supportive and can counsel young people and their parents about sexuality issues.
3) Be sure your programs are in the referral systems of local congregations. Introduce yourself and your services at a local clergy meeting or mail letters to local congregations describing your programs. Ask if you can have your pamphlets posted on bulletin boards or available in the foyers or social halls. Volunteer to do programs in your area of expertise.
4) Offer to do training programs or workshops for the clergy and the religious educators in your community. Know what is being taught about sexuality in your community congregations and offer to train the leaders or teach certain sessions. Offer to co-sponsor programs at faith-based communities for parents, young people and adults.
5) In your classroom programs, be sure to identify the diversity of religious points of views on controversial issues. The Guidelines For Comprehensive Sexuality Education includes religion as one of 37 recommended topics. Remember that religion is not

monolithic on these issues. Help young people explore the influences on their attitudes and behaviors.
6) In clinic counseling, explore your clients' religious beliefs and their involvement in a religious community. A girl who is disaffected at school may find meaning being part of a faith community. Answers to these types of questions may give us insight into their behaviors as well as their risk factors.

The Religious Institute on Sexual Morality, Justice and Healing is a forum for progressive religious leaders to join together to advocate not just for sexuality education for young people but for sexual justice in denominations and faith communities as well as in society. More than 2,200 clergy, theologians and religious educators from 35 denominations have endorsed the "Religious Declaration on Sexual Morality, Justice and Healing" since it was published in January 2000. The declaration calls for a sexual ethic focused on personal relationships and social justice rather than on particular sexual acts or the age, marital status or sexual orientation of the participants. The declaration urges religious leaders and faith communities to provide comprehensive sexuality education, advocate for sexual and reproductive rights and assure the full inclusion of women and sexual minorities in congregational life, denominations and society at large.

There is a compelling need for religious voices to join together to offer prophetic witness to God's good gift of sexuality to all people. Our ministry is to heal the brokenness that so many experience about their sexuality and to help people celebrate their sexuality with holiness and integrity. We must be committed to helping young people understand their sexual development and offer them the skills for moral discernment and responsible decision-making. We must offer all people the opportunity and the ability to choose meaningful, intimate relationships that are based on consent, mutuality, honesty and responsibility.

Portions of this chapter have been adapted from previous works, including the Rev. Debra W. Haffner, "A Time to Build: Creating Sexuality Healthy Faith Communities" (CT: Religious Institute on Sexual Morality, Justice, and Healing, 2002) and Haffner's "Teens and Sex: Just Say . . . What?" in Body and Soul (Cleveland: The Pilgrim Press, 2002.)

The Rev. Debra W. Haffner, MPH, M.Div., is director of the Religious Institute on Sexual Morality, Justice and Healing. She was president of the Sexuality Information and Education Council of the United States from 1988 to 2000. An ordained Unitarian Universalist minister, she has been a sexuality educator for 28 years and is the author of two award-winning books for parents on raising sexually healthy children and teenagers.

Adapted from
The Sex Lives of Teenagers

By Lynn Ponton, M.D.
Author, Professor and Psychiatrist

"**H**ealthy sexual life." Few parents are able to say the words, let alone acknowledge that this is one of their aspirations for their child.

In a culture that offers few rituals to its adolescents to mark their passage into adulthood, teens seek out and create their own. Engaging in risky behavior is one way that many teens define their own identity and create their own rituals. In a country where half of teens have sex at age 16 or younger, and three-quarters by 19, the initiation of sexual intercourse has become a rite of passage.

Often, peers are the witnesses for the sexual initiatives, helping with preparations and hearing the stories afterward, but mothers play an increasingly important role with daughters. Two separate studies have shown they are vital in the formation of gender-role identity for girls, as well as body image, two crucial aspects of sexual identity.

In the halls of middle schools and high schools, girls and boys are being pressured to become sexually active. Among the inducements used are "Everyone's doing it," "You're frigid," "Be a man . . ." Written down, they don't seem particularly threatening. It is different when you hear them directed at you by a boyfriend or girlfriend or by peers. Under those circumstances, they can leave you tongue-tied and doubting yourself.

A teen's peer group plays a strong role in determining his or her attitudes about sex and sexual behavior through the information and misinformation they provide, as well as the values they transmit. Parents also play a role in relaying their values, and a somewhat more-limited role in transmitting information on the specifics of sexual behavior. Much sexual information is communicated nonverbally as teens watch and imitate their parents' sexual behavior. Parents often do not know what to tell their children about sex because they either lack information or are unsure of their own values. Fathers have been found to be particularly uninvolved in the sexuality education of their children. Parents frequently deal with sexual matters with a single retort or threat instead of taking part in an ongoing dialogue. There are many reasons parents have difficulty talking to their kids, including embarrassment, fears that a sexually explicit conversation will provoke teen sexual activity or the absence or lack of a parental or peer support format. Taboo undoubtedly plays a strong role. Talking about sex is itself a sexual interaction, and as such, its avoidance may be part of the incest taboo.

Ongoing conversations are one of the best ways to address sex with children and teens and can, over time, help to minimize the taboo and discomfort for both generations alike.

One of the most important things that I have learned from working with teens is that their sexual patterns are extremely diverse. Yet teens feel acute pressure to be sexually "normal," whatever that is, and struggle to make their own behavior fit into what they imagine fits that pattern. They keep much of their sexual lives hidden. There is often a story to share, though, and they are looking for someone to listen. Their reluctance to talk about sexual matters is combined with social taboos, and the result is that they learn very little about what teenage sexual experiences are really like. Into this gap, television, movies and music videos slide with dramatic stories that make it appear as if all teens are not only participating, but also adept at sexual intercourse. This often infuriates parents, who view the media as aggressively seducing their children long before they are ready. The media's aggressive use of teenage sexuality to sell everything may infuriate parents, but it is more demanding to teens themselves who are struggling to find out exactly what is "normal" and if they are included.

Fifty percent of America's 16-year-olds are having sexual intercourse, a figure that is actually lower than those in many developed countries. The United States excels in one area, however, that of dangerous sexual risk-taking—i.e., unprotected sexual intercourse resulting in unwanted pregnancy and sexually transmitted diseases. For generations, this country has struggled with adolescent risk-taking of all types. American culture is defined by risk-taking—the successful pursuit of the American Dream virtually requires it—but we are not a society particularly adept at risk assessment.

The general attitude about risk-taking is only one factor that contributes to higher rates of sexual risk-taking, however. Attitudes about sexuality also play an important role. Our culture is plagued with conflict about how to handle sexuality. Parts of this country are extremely restrictive, discouraging masturbation, homosexuality and even adolescent sex, and labeling them as crimes, sins or sickness. Adults try to discourage young people from becoming sexually active by lecturing them about the virtues of virginity, by not openly discussing sexual matters and by making it difficult for teens to obtain contraception. Yet as conservatives criticize teen sexuality, the United States is not by any means a sexually permissive culture, despite the idealized and very disturbed views of teenage sexuality in the media. If anything, the United States is a fairly restrictive sexual culture characterized by strong taboos, poor communication and restrictive gender roles. We do not give a consistent message about sexuality.

Because teens struggle to discover their sexuality in a culture that is giving them a highly conflicted message, it is a tribute to their energy and power that many are able to develop healthy sexual lives. Many, sadly, are not. Sexual education efforts in this country are paralyzed by these same conflicts. Many states insist on abstinence-based sex education efforts and do not allow access to contraception. Teens' views of their sexuality, however, differ from those of adults. For teens, the ways of sex are fraught with struggle, but also filled with excitement and pleasure.

I have had the opportunity to speak with hundreds of teens about what their sexuality means to them. Some answered that it made them feel lovable or more adult. Some described intense physical pleasure. Some told how it nurtured intimacy with another person, fulfilled a desire to become pregnant, promoted status in his or her peer group or allowed for a surrender to desire or to another person. For some, it brought relief from boredom or escape from life's pressures or an opportunity to test out biological equipment. For others, it involved re-enactments of a sexually traumatic event from the past or was useful as a tool for barter in obtaining money or material goods. Some characterized it as an expected part of a current relationship, a representation of "true love," a useful weapon or a personal expression of growth and spirituality.

The sexual culture of the United States is not only confused, alternating its messages between restrictive and permissive, but violent as well. Violent sexual images often are transmitted through the media, but teens experience this violence in other ways, too. Teens struggling with their sexual identity or orientation fear that violence will be directed at them if they deviate from the norm. This affects all teens because at some point every teen feels that he or she is sexually different and fears reprisal. The narrow gender and sexual orientation norms affect all teens, not only girls who were sexually active at early ages or boys who believe that they are gay. Narrow gender roles force a macho identity on boys who are striving to become men in a patriarchal culture. Boys feel the pressure to rapidly acquire experience and become sexual experts, to have penises that are powerful. The culture reinforces and rewards this. For girls, the message is more contradictory. On the one hand, they, too, are encouraged to become powerful with their sexuality, told explicitly and implicitly to use it as their main source of control. On the other hand, girls who do this often are cast out as sluts. The double standard continues. Teens of both sexes are fearful as they struggle to develop and understand their sexual orientation. Frightened of their own feelings and the culture's reaction, some scapegoat others. Many adults encourage this attitude. Tolerance and understanding of sexual diversity are too little discussed or understood.

Teens are sexually active everywhere—most commonly in their homes. Before we find out where teens are doing what sexually, we need to be able to both listen and talk with them about sexuality. Many parents know that they should prepare themselves to guide their child through the teen years, but when they think about sex, they shut down. Rather than letting embarrassment paralyze them, it should act as a clue, helping parents detect what they are afraid of. In talking with teens about sex, it is important to be direct, use simple language and admit to your own embarrassment. In general, teens don't like jokes about sex unless they are telling them so begin slowly in this area. The discussions need to start long before the child is a teenager. Some ideas for earlier discussions include biological information, identifying and exploring language a child may learn outside the home and observing and discussing messages around sexuality in the media. It is preferable for parents to talk about feelings and lessons they've learned through experience without disclosing specific personal details. Exploring stories about other teens—real or fictional—also can promote discussion. Ask teens for their opinions; don't just give them yours. Educate yourself about the spectrum of adolescent sexual behaviors. Enforcing rigid gender roles or sexual orientation can be extremely damaging. The wise parent recognizes that adolescence is about taking risks, sexually and in other ways, and will want his or her teen to have safe, healthy options, even if this means engaging in activity that runs counter to parental values.

All teenagers have sexual lives, whether with others or through fantasies, and an important part of adolescence is thinking about and experimenting with aspects of sexuality. This helps adolescents discover and develop their individual sexual identity, which is more than sexual orientation. Encouraging your teen to talk with other trusted adults about sexuality is also important.

Parents communicate values and morals best by example, so be aware of how you speak and act concerning sexual and gender issues in front of your teens, who are watching, whether they acknowledge it or not. They respond best to suggestions rather than directives, highlighting the importance of the parent's role as guide during these crucial years.

The imperatives around knowing more about teen sexuality extend to the culture at large as well. Parents should find out what sexuality education their children and teens are learning in school, and what they are not learning. Many teachers will welcome parental input. There are other sources of sexual education besides school. Many youth organizations for girls and boys offer programs. Health care providers such as pediatricians, specialists in adolescent medicine, child and adolescent psychiatrists, psychologists or social workers are familiar with programs and are available for individual consultation also.

Helping society understand this taboo and complex subject may seem overwhelming. Educating yourself and your child is an important place to start, but it is largely uncharted territory. Conversations about these important subjects are unusual enough among adults so it is not surprising that they are even more rare between adults and teens. Adults have to start these conversations.

If you listen openly to your teen's own stories to learn about their hopes for and struggles with sex and offer them guidance without being authoritarian, you will have gone a long way toward helping them develop their own healthy outlook on their sexual lives and fostering the risk-assessment skills they'll need along the way.

From *The Sex Lives of Teenagers*

by Lynn Ponton, © 2000 by Lynn Ponton. Used by permission of Dutton, a division of Penguin Group (USA) Inc.

Lynn Ponton, M.D. is a leading figure in adolescent psychiatry, with more than 20 years of experience working with teenagers and their parents. She is a professor of child and adolescent psychiatry at the University of California, San Francisco. Dr. Ponton is the author of two books addressing teen sexuality and risk-taking.

Understanding the Concept of Sexuality from a Medical Perspective

**By Barbara Staggers, M.D.,
Chief of Adolescent Medicine
Children's Hospital and Research Center,
Oakland, California**

Sexuality is a term that is culturally specific. How sexuality is expressed (i.e., what constitutes a healthy or unhealthy individual) is influenced by factors such as spiritual, ethical, cultural and moral concern[1]. Although in the United States today there is public and professional consensus about what is unhealthy sexually for adolescents[2] (with large bodies of research documenting morbidities associated with adolescent sexual practices), there is limited public and professional consensus about what is sexually healthy for adolescents. Sexuality encompasses more than just sexual behaviors, preferences or identity. Its broad range of definitions varies depending upon language, community and culture. For the purposes of this chapter, I propose the following definition of sexuality:

> "Human sexuality is a term that encompasses the sexual knowledge, beliefs, attitudes, values and

behaviors of individuals. Its dimensions include: identity, orientation, roles and personality; thoughts, feelings and relationships; and the anatomy, physiology and biochemistry of the sexual response system."

The concept of a healthy sexuality throughout the life span has developed with clear definitions of sexually related terminology (listed as additional references at the end of the book). Within this construct, sexuality is seen as a natural and healthy part of life with human beings being inherently sexual. Thus, sexuality is experienced and expressed in distinct ways dependent upon the stage of the life cycle (i.e., infancy, childhood, adolescence, adulthood). It is within this framework that the concept of a sexually healthy adolescent can be explored.

The achievement of a healthy adolescent sexuality is a key developmental task. The sexuality that evolves during childhood and adolescence lays the foundation for adult sexual health and intimacy. In order to have an understanding of the process of adolescent development as it pertains to sexuality, it is important to have a clear understanding of the stages of development.

Adolescence is a time of dynamic transition from childhood to adulthood. It is not continuous nor a uniformly synchronous process[3]. An integral feature of this transition is developing a satisfactory sexual identity[4]. Sexual development involves integration of gender roles, self-concept, body image, emotions, relationships, religious beliefs, societal norms as well as intercourse and other sexual behaviors[5]. It is widely accepted that teenagers must complete six developmental tasks in order to become healthy adults. These tasks include physical and sexual maturation, autonomy/independence, conceptual identity,[6] functional identity,[7] cognitive development and sexual self-concept.[8] All of the tasks are attained within the three developmental stages of adolescent development.

The three fundamental stages of adolescence overlap tremendously among teens as they emerge into adulthood. They include early, middle and late adolescence. Early adolescence occurs at approximately 10-13 years of age and is a time of rapid physical change. Although the complete process of the physical changes that occurs during this stage is beyond the scope of this chapter, it is important to recognize how these changes require psychosocial adjustment on the part of the adolescent, family and other adults[9]. Young girls are entering puberty at younger ages than in the past. Currently, over the last three decades, the average age of menarche is 12-12.5 years. There are ethnic differences, with African American girls entering puberty earlier than Caucasians[10]. Consequently, entering puberty earlier has seen an increase in sexual experimentation, including intercourse. Both sexes who experience earlier pubertal development are more likely to have had sexual intercourse. Yet boys still lag behind girls in pubertal maturation. Young girls tend to seek older partners, which can increase the risk of sexual exploitation.

There is a preoccupation with self but an uncertainty with appearance and attractiveness. As a result, the teen has an increased interest in sexual anatomy and outcomes of puberty, for instance menstruation, breast development and masturbation. Girls often develop a feeling of being center stage with everyone noting her physical transformation. Sexual experimentation can occur in this stage, but sexual intercourse (vaginal, anal) is less common. Boys tend to initiate sexual intercourse but not on a regular basis. Girls are much more likely to delay intercourse as an early adolescent. When contact is made with peers of the opposite sex, it usually is in a group of friends. Same-sex relationships can be strongly emotional, and there may be homosexual exploration.

Young adolescents are concrete thinkers and see the world as black or white. The concrete thinking process contributes to the lack of projecting themselves into the future. Consequently, they cannot perceive long-range implications of current decisions. In addition, young people are trying to achieve autonomy from their parents. Thus, independence-dependence struggles occur between the adolescent and the parent or parental figures. In some instances, the conflicts can create emotional voids because of the separation from the parent, and behavioral problems may arise.

It is important to note that youth from disadvantaged communities may not get the support for developing a healthy identity and may find other ways to foster these feelings, for example drug use and sexual experimentation. Yet in all groups, sexual behaviors may be a reflection of peer norms, independence-dependence struggles and an inability to control impulses regardless of long-term consequences.[12]

Middle adolescence occurs from 14 to 16 years of age. Physical changes are almost complete, and teens become more comfortable with their bodies. Much time is spent making the body more attractive. Abstract thought begins to develop in this stage along with feelings of omnipotence and invincibility. There is a new ability to examine the feelings of others, which can foster closer relationships with peers. Greater autonomy also occurs and coupled with omniscient feelings can contribute to risk-taking behaviors and a belief that they cannot be harmed. This is important in the context of unintentional pregnancies and sexually transmitted infections that are prevalent in this stage. As the teen increases his or her separation from the parents, peer groups begin to become important guiding forces in behaviors. The peer group affirms the teen's self-image. Sexual energy is at a high level, and there is an emphasis in physical contact. Middle adolescents develop the ability to fall in love. Dating is common, including making out (petting) during this stage of development. Also casual relationships with coital and noncoital contacts are common in an exploratory and exploitative nature.

Late adolescence, 17 to 21 years old, is characterized by full physical maturation. A more adult role is taken on, which includes understanding abstract thoughts and concepts. Sexuality is more expressive and less exploitative, and as a result, intimate relationships may develop. There is an understanding of the consequences of actions. Yet the cognitive and emotional level, along with developmental age, influence sexual decision-making, in particular contraceptive choices and sexually transmitted infection prevention. Family dynamics change to a more adult relationship with parents and peer groups not as important to the young adult as they were in middle adolescence. Uncertainty in sexual orientation decreases with chronological age. Most late adolescents are sure of their sexual orientation. One caveat is gay and lesbian youth, which may not "come out" until later adulthood.

Adolescent sexuality is an important developmental process. The young person has to accomplish many developmental tasks in order to have a productive adulthood and a healthy sexuality. Health professionals, politicians and parents must realize that all teenagers are sexual beings whether they are sexually active or not. Furthermore, society should recognize that adolescents have sexual experiences and educational strategies, and support must be provided in order to confer the skills necessary for healthy relationship decisions.

A young person has to accomplish many developmental tasks in order to realize a productive adulthood and a healthy sexuality. Achieving sexual health requires the integration of many factors (i.e. physical, psychological, economic, spiritual, cultural, educational). It also encompasses normal development and reproductive health and a combination of skills and characteristics.

The current available research in the area of adolescent sexuality focuses primarily on sexual behaviors and outcomes. Few studies have examined the context of adolescent romantic relationships and noncoital behaviors (although there is a growing body of work in this area). There is a need to continue to expand the diversity of the research populations to include groups other than Caucasians and African Americans. Available data have traditionally focused on heterosexual intercourse and contraceptive use. This data does not adequately describe the wide range of sexual behaviors practiced by adolescents today—physical acts such as handholding; kissing; masturbation; touching; caressing; oral, vaginal and anal intercourse and oral genital contact. Research has not yet adequately explored the full range of factors that influence a healthy sexuality especially as young people have evolved over the past 60 years. The exploration of this broader concept of sexuality is important because adolescents comprise about 15 percent of the population, and nearly half (45.6 percent) of high school students have had sexual intercourse. To date, most public debate has focused on which sexual behaviors are appropriate for adolescents and ignored the complex dimensions of sexuality.

The dialogue and controversy surrounding a sexually healthy adolescent is never more evident than in the growing exploration of research on the gay, lesbian, transsexual, transvestite, queer and questioning youth. Whether the adolescent is bisexual, homosexual or heterosexual is all within the range of normal within the sexually healthy adolescent theoretical construct. Confusion surrounding terminology; issues such as discrimination, sexism and prejudice; and increasing the knowledge base regarding sexual practices have moved to the forefront.[15]

Homosexuality is a difficult issue for adolescents and their families. To further complicate things, the term "homosexual," often replaced with "gay," has failed to include the range of sexual expression that can be encountered by health professionals and the community. "Queer" has lost much of its derogatory sting to become an inclusive term to describe the full range of sexual expression. This includes gay referring to homosexual males or females, "lesbian" referring to homosexual females, "bisexual" referring to those sexually attracted to people of both sexes, "transgender" as an umbrella term referring to "transsexuals" (preoperative, postoperative, and a desire to have no surgery, but may or may not be taking hormones to alter their physical appearance), "transvestites" (cross-dressers who are not necessarily gay) and "drag artists" (male or female impersonators). And "questioning" is a term referring to those who are unsure of their stance on the continuum of sexual orientation. Another useful collective term combining the first letter of each of these words is "GLBTQ."

To help understand homosexual and GLBTQ identity development, it is useful to examine the Troiden model of identity development. Troiden[16] postulated a four-stage model. Stage 1 is Sensitization; there are often feelings of being different from peers. Stage 2, Identity Confusion, is same-sex arousal, and this can cause confusion prompting behaviors such as denial and avoidance. Stage 3, Identity Assumption, is self-identity as a GLBTQ, sexual experimentation and investigation of the subculture. And in stage 4, Commitment, there is identity acceptance leading to an emotional and sexual GLBTQ relationship. The progression of these stages is not always linear, may be different for ethnic minorities[17] and can be complicated by high-risk behaviors.

Internalization of society's homophobia can be a contributing factor of depression and suicide, abuse of drugs and alcohol, school failure, sexually transmitted diseases because of risky sexual behavior and eating disorders. An adolescent, who discloses his or her sexual orientation, may be vulnerable to verbal and physical harassment at school and home.[18] This withdrawal of support especially at home can result in homelessness and survival sex.

The overall goal of the of work of the health care provider is to provide a nonjudgmental and safe environment that permits the GLBTQ adolescent to seek routine health care.[19] The adept health professional should be aware of local outreach agencies, support groups and role models in the community permitting a holistic approach to care of the GLBTQ adolescent. Just as in any area of adolescent sexual health, the culture of sexual wellness of the adolescent must be explored.

Barbara Staggers, M.D. is chief of adolescent medicine for Children's Hospital & Research Center in Oakland, California.

Lessons from Abroad: Strategies to Promote European Approaches to Adolescent Sexuality

**By Barbara Huberman, RN, BSN, MeD,
Director of Education and Outreach
Advocates for Youth**

The United States has one of the highest teen birthrates and teen sexually transmitted disease (STD) rates among industrialized nations. Researchers, program providers, policymakers, prevention advocates and educators have struggled for many years to determine how to reduce these rates in America.

One answer is to look to other nations. Three countries in particular—the Netherlands, Germany and France—have policies and practices that have contributed to reducing and maintaining low teen birth and STD rates.

Adolescent sexual health indicators in the three European countries far outshine those in the United States. For instance, the U.S. adolescent birthrate (49 per 1,000) is nine times higher than that of the Netherlands, almost five times higher than the rate in France and nearly four times higher than in Germany.[1,2] The teen abortion rate in the United States (27.5 per 1,000) is nearly eight times higher than the rate in Germany, over seven times higher than in the Netherlands and nearly three times higher than the rate in France.[3,4] In the United States, the teen gonorrhea rate is over 74 times higher than in the Netherlands and France.[5]

Welfare benefits in the three European countries are also much higher than in the United States, social support systems such as national health plans are more comprehensive and cost less and sexuality education for young people is a priority.

Finally, in the United States, teens begin having sexual intercourse at the same age or a younger age than teens in the other three nations, and American teens have more partners.[6]

Since 1995, Advocates for Youth and the University of North Carolina at Charlotte have sponsored a national institute each summer to enhance the knowledge and skills of youth risk-behavior professionals in this country. In 1998, the institute became an international study tour designed to familiarize American professionals in the sexual health field with programs and policies in selected European countries. Since 1998, more than 200 participants, including masters and doctoral students, prevention advocates, educators, state and national leaders, funders, health care providers, authors and program providers have been selected to visit the three European countries for two weeks each summer.

In an effort to have a more direct impact on American state policies and programs, the institute selects and supports teams of experts from a targeted number of states, including those directly responsible for developing strategies and policies. These teams also receive follow-up support from Advocates for Youth.

In each of the European countries, the group visits clinics, agencies and prevention organizations. Lecturers, researchers, media experts, government officials, educators and health professionals offer critical analyses of policy, culture, religion and strategic interventions to reduce sexual risk-taking behaviors. Participants also conduct informal street interviews with young people and parents.

After the first study tour, various key topics, including sexuality education, family and community relations, religion and public values, media and access to health services became the basis for a monograph "European Approaches to Adolescent Sexual Behavior and Responsibility." It included how to create relevant programs and policies that support the rights of young people to education and services that protect them from unplanned pregnancy, STDs and HIV. In 1999, a documentary video was produced along with a new monograph on the impact and influence of religion on adolescent reproductive sexual health. It has been a fruitful experience for participants and sheds light on the problems as well as potential solutions for the United States.

Lessons Learned

There are numerous lessons to be learned from these three nations—lessons that add up to a better approach to sexual health.

Dutch, German, and French adults view adolescent sexual development as a normal and healthy part of biological, social, emotional and cultural development. Sexuality education focuses on informed choice and sexual responsibility for all members of the society, including adolescents. These nations focus on safer-sex messages rather than dictates about the morality of premarital sex or homosexual relations. Public campaigns coordinate with school sexuality education, condom and contraceptive access and nonjudgmental attitudes from adults to promote sexual health. Educators and administrators in these three nations prohibit no topics being discussed, and teachers are free to teach as they see fit. No topic is too controversial if young people want to discuss it.

Public and private schools in the Netherlands and Germany acknowledge that sexuality education is important and concentrate most heavily in middle and secondary years. While sexuality education is taught as a specific health unit in Germany and France, it is also widely integrated wherever it is relevant—in courses on literature, languages, social studies, religion, sciences or current events. And the teaching is generally a collaborative effort among school personnel, community youth workers, reproductive health clinicians, parents and communities.

The three European governments also support broad, consistent and long-term public education campaigns that use of television, radio, billboards, nightclubs, pharmacies and doctors, among others, in the dissemination of safe-sex messages. There, the media are viewed as a potential solution, not as a problem. And given the recent debate in the United States on the role of the media in sending inappropriate messages about sexuality to minors, it's interesting to note that in the three European nations, there appears to be little concern about sexually explicit media. This may be because there is more open, honest and consistent communication about sexuality between adults and teens through the media, schools, families and health providers. In contrast to the United States, public policies to reduce pregnancies, abortions and STDs in the three countries are research-driven, with little influence from religious or political groups. These societies do not embrace or promote the concept of abstinence until marriage.

In Europe, being a partner in an intimate sexual relationship, especially for older adolescents, is perceived as normal and natural and a positive and healthy component of maturation. Completing an education and attaining economic self-sufficiency are the norms before marriage and having children.

National health insurance in the three countries also gives sexually active youth free and convenient access to contraception, including emergency contraception. The goal is to reduce abortions and STDs. As a result, young people generally believe it is irresponsible to not use protection. To most European teens, it is always, "safe sex or no sex." Although teen condom use there is fairly consistent with teen condom use in the United States, major differences emerge when comparing teen use of other effective means of contraception. In the Netherlands, nearly 67 percent of sexually active adolescent females use oral contraceptives, and about 63 percent of sexually active adolescent females in Germany report using oral contraceptives. By contrast, 20.5 percent of sexually active adolescent females in the United States report using oral contraceptives.

Advocated for Youth learned that in the three European countries, parents and communities accept youth as sexual beings and accept sexual intercourse as a logical outcome in intimate relationships. Most adults in these three nations do not see teenage sex as a problem as long as teens use protection. Parents in the Netherlands, Germany and France want young people to develop a healthy sexuality and support both abstinent and sexually active teens in making responsible decisions. Dutch, German and French parents use multiple channels to ensure that teens are well informed and socially skilled and may provide teens with condoms and contraception to protect themselves. Parents then trust teens to make good choices for themselves and to be responsible. The argument in America against such a comprehensive program is that it will encourage sexual activity among teens, but the research and practice in Europe suggests otherwise.

Educational institutions can play a critical role in helping the United States to achieve similar success in supporting young people to delay the initiation of first sexual intercourse and use condoms and contraception to reduce pregnancy and STD rates.

Before the 1990s, there was only a small minority who tried to prevent schools from providing any services or educational programs that enhance sexual health and well-being. Even then, it was clear the American public felt strongly that schools needed to educate young people about sexuality. Critics of formal sexuality education programs began to attack existing programs and demand, in the name of "family values," that programs and curricula teach nothing but abstinence until marriage. They also encouraged using fear, shame and guilt rather than facts—as if believing that young people can't be trusted to make healthy and safe decisions with factual information. Competent sexuality educators were, and still are, attacked as immoral promoters of sexual promiscuity. As large, conservative, powerful organizations, both secular and religious, got involved, pressure was put on Congress in 1997 to include a $250 million appropriation to states that funds programs that exclusively teach abstinence until marriage while withholding safe-sex information. Additional millions have been added each year since 1997.

Programs supported with these funds in all states—except California, which refused the funds—must tell young people that the only appropriate sex is sex within marriage and those who engage in premarital sex are acting immorally and will suffer physical and psychological damage. Needless to say, no research supports these claims.

Scientific research and the Western European experience show that providing information to young people about sex does not cause them to have sex. Openness and honesty do not lead to promiscuity—they lead to young people respecting themselves and behaving responsibly to a greater degree. It is clear; adults can encourage and support young people to choose abstinence in their early teen years, while encouraging and supporting sexually active youth to protect themselves by using condoms and contraception.

Our vision is to help build a society in which:

- Adolescents have the **Right** to balanced, accurate and realistic sexuality education, confidential and affordable health services and a secure stake in the future.
- Youth have **Respect.** Today, they are perceived only as the problem. Valuing young people means they are part of the solution and are included in the development of programs and policies that affect their well-being.
- Society has the **Responsibility** to provide young people with the tools they need to safeguard their sexual health, and young people have the **Responsibility** to protect themselves from too early childbearing and sexually transmitted infections, including HIV.

This trilogy of values underpins the social philosophy of adolescent sexual and reproductive health in the Netherlands, Germany and France. The following are recommendations for schools, health professionals, religious leaders, the media and prevention advocates seeking to create this approach.

Policies and Laws

- Modify policies and laws to encourage both abstinent behavior (particularly in young and middle adolescents) and protective sexual behavior in all sexually active people, including adolescents.
- Revise the national "abstinence until marriage" legislation to include abstinence and protective sexual behavior (safe sex or no sex). Attach quasi-experimental evaluation components to each so that the behavioral effectiveness can be determined in the United States.
- Fund the development of ongoing, national, strategic sexually transmitted infection and pregnancy

prevention efforts based on research. Adopt policies based on this research, without political, religious or other extraneous influences.
- Maintain anonymous and confidential testing, and remove any parental consent requirements for accessing preventive services.
- Support ongoing research on adolescent health data, program evaluation and behavior change.

Reproductive Health Services

- Develop and modify health services and resources to assist adolescents in maintaining sexual health and protective sexual behavior.
- Implement policies or conditions that significantly remove barriers for adolescents to receive basic health care and reproductive health care.
- Provide oral contraceptives and other medical methods of contraception to women under age 20 without a PAP smear or pelvic exam. (The U.S. Food and Drug Administration has removed the requirement for a PAP smear and pelvic exam to receive birth control pills, but many providers still demand it.)
- Reduce initial intake paperwork to a minimum (one page), make directions simple and information requested noninvasive.
- Provide youth-friendly services (phone inquiries, appointments, receptions, separate waiting room from adults).
- Provide services at youth friendly hours (3 to 8 p.m., weekends and holidays).
- Provide low cost or nominal cost services.
- Establish one-stop shopping for education, counseling and services addressing a variety of health needs.
- Improve access to condoms and contraception for all sexually active people.

- Lower by national subsidy, the prices of condoms.
- Provide and maintain condom dispensaries in youth-designated locations.
- Increase knowledge about and access to emergency contraception (EC).
- Place EC messages on answering machines of reproductive health service telephones.
- Develop media campaigns for EC targeting older adolescents through college campus newspapers, health centers, health occupations, professional practice and medical education programs.
- Provide articles and advertisements with 1-800-NOT-2-LATE for EC in age-appropriate media (teen magazines, etc.).
- Expand and fund school-based clinics that include reproductive health care.
- Mandate reproductive health services as a part of coverage in national health insurance plans for all women. Provide coverage for school-age children through school-based health insurance.

Sexuality Education

- Provide age-appropriate and developmentally appropriate sexuality education for children in schools within the context of comprehensive health education and other relevant courses.
- Provide honest, realistic and developmentally appropriate sexuality education programs, resources and training.
- Borrow, develop and modify sexuality education curricula based on input derived from student-needs assessments, student focus groups and student questions.
- Fund the training of teachers to become knowledgeable

and comfortable in soliciting and answering student questions about sexuality issues appropriately and honestly.
- Through school counselors and school social workers, identify youth who need education and support at earlier or later ages than their peers and provide appropriate programming and resources for them.
- Normalize sexuality as a part of being human. Focus on positive aspects of human sexuality as well as preventing negative consequences.
- Integrate discussion of sexuality with other relevant subjects in the comprehensive health education program (drug education, community health, communicable diseases, social health) and in other courses such as biology, social studies, literature, etc., as appropriate.
- Develop or borrow model lessons, resources and training that frame sexuality within the universal values of love, committed relationships, choice, respect and responsibility.
- Increase opportunities for career development, educational opportunity and job training in schools.
- Integrate community efforts for prevention into the school sexuality education curriculum.
- Integrate educational components of national and local media campaigns.
- Integrate information about local prevention services.
- Integrate activities about local community, youth-development projects.
- Increase teacher training in sexuality education
- Enable school districts and regional associations of independent and private schools to provide ongoing training and support for sexuality education instruction as a part of comprehensive school health education.

Mass Media

- Provide ongoing, annual national campaigns to promote protective behaviors in all-age sexually active Americans, including adolescents.
- Provide funds for annually targeted nationwide campaigns that are strategically planned, based on research, utilize social marketing and learning theories for protective behavior and are disseminated widely through a variety of channels (magazines, cinemas, clubs, television, schools, posters, billboards, physician offices, pharmacies, CD-ROM, PSAs, Web sites, etc.).
- Create public and private partnerships for airtime, space and distribution of mass media messages.
- Provide tax incentives for television and cinema to depict sexuality and sexual behavior in a more realistic and protective manner.
- Invite youth into the process of developing adolescent-targeted, mass media campaigns; employ teens as the message carriers.
- Develop specialty campaigns around holidays, spring breaks, prom seasons, etc.

Family and Community

- Assist families and communities in communication with young people about sexuality and related developmental issues; provide family and community resources for adolescent growth and development including support for abstinence and protective sexual behavior.
- Shift the paradigm by stimulating a national discussion about treating young people as a valuable asset and a national resource.
- Teach/role model with parents and adults how to be available, nonjudgmental listeners and resources for youth.

- Teach/role model with parents and adults how to communicate early, openly, honestly and realistically about sex.
- Educate parents and adults to respect youth as individuals who make choices.
- Enable parents and adults to acknowledge sexuality as a normal developmental process.
- Help parents and adults give young people increasing measures of trust and responsibility.
- Provide opportunities and incentives for parenting education, parent/youth education and communication about sexuality.
- Assist and support youth-serving organizations to include abstinence and protective sexual behavior in programming as a part of funding requirements.
- Engage youth through focus groups and in advisory capacities in planning youth programs as a part of funding requirements.

Religion and Values

- Develop a proactive national agenda to reconcile religious doctrine with sexuality as a human quality. Express public support for abstinence and protection as hierarchical values for sexual health in society.
- Support public health policies including both abstinence and protective sexual behavior for sexually active people prior to or outside of marriage.
- Develop avenues and programs for addressing sexuality with young people including committed relationships, responsibility, respect, choice, abstinence and protection behaviors.
- Explore positive themes and messages about sexuality in sermons, classes, programs and activities.
- Train clergy, youth ministers, educators and lay leaders

in communicating about sexuality with all ages of the congregation.
- Engage the support of community spiritual leaders to speak out in support of sexuality education programs in the schools or community.

Barbara Huberman, R.N., BSN, MeD is the national director of education and outreach for Advocates for Youth in Washington, D.C., and the coordinator of the Rights. Respect. Responsibility. National Campaign. Ms. Huberman was a founding board member of the National Campaign to Prevent Teen Pregnancy, as well as a past president of the National Organization on Adolescent Pregnancy, Parenting and Prevention.

Epilogue

It is impossible to take a truly comprehensive look at teenage pregnancy prevention and teen birthrates without addressing an emotional topic that tends to polarize adults: abortion.

Because the purpose of this book is to increase awareness among opinion leaders and policymakers about successful approaches to preventing unplanned pregnancy among adolescents, we chose not to include a chapter that specifically addresses abortion. After all, if one can help a young person successfully avoid an unplanned pregnancy, abortion isn't necessary. That in and of itself should be one of the primary reasons that abortion foes support a comprehensive, realistic approach to teen pregnancy prevention.

Having said that, we will use the opportunity in this epilogue to give the reader a brief insight into this issue, hopefully to encourage further study on the topic in order to fully understand the complete picture when discussing teenage pregnancy prevention.

Dr. Jocelyn M. Elders, former surgeon general of the United States, has this to say: "In America, we are in the midst of a sexual crisis. We lead the Western world in virtually every sexual problem: teenage pregnancy, abortion, rape, incest, child abuse, sexually transmitted disease, HIV/AIDS and many more. Yet when the surgeon general issues a call to action on sexual health urging comprehensive sex education, abstinence and other measures to promote responsible sexual behavior, we want to fire the surgeon general."

She also states: "Treating sex as dangerous is dangerous in itself. We need to be matter-of-fact about what is, after all, a fact of life." Dr. Elders suggests that parents and other adults involved in young people's lives read *Harmful to Minors: The Perils of Protecting Children from Sex,* by Judith Levine to become educated about the facts about adolescent sexuality, including abortion, among young people. In the book's foreword, Elders continues her statements by saying: "Judith Levine argues convincingly that there is an intimate connection between the values we display in our sexual lives and the values we display as a society. She is right—sex is a moral issue, but not in the way the Christian right claims. Children must be taught sexual ethics and responsibility, inside and outside the home, just as they are taught how to behave in any number of public and private arenas. Teaching children to have self-respect, to feel good about themselves, to make good decisions—to me, that is sexuality education."

Levine addresses the subject of abortion in a chapter in *Harmful to Minors* aptly titled, "Compulsory Motherhood." "Considering the clamor it has raised," she writes, "the anti-choice movement has achieved a monumental and paradoxical triumph in the decades after Roe: *it has wrought a near-total public silence on the subject of abortion in the discourse of teen sex.*" Contrasting this situation with that in "most developed countries, (where) the surgical termination of a pregnancy is a legal, normal, part of women's reproductive lives," Levine argues that American anti-choice activism "has transformed the emotional and moral conception of abortion no less than the practicalities of getting one." Three decades after legalization, "one can hardly speak of abortion without a note of deep misgiving or regret – if one speaks of it at all...What this means for unmarried teens is that unwanted pregnancy has regained its age-old resonance of sin and doom, and motherhood again has come to feel like the near-inevitable price of sexual pleasure." The atmosphere of silence, shame and fear affects not only opponents of abortion, Levine says, but also supporters of reproductive choice and comprehensive sexuality education.

Health experts point out that it is necessary to acknowledge that the decline in births to teens has been, in part, due to the increase in abortion rates among teenagers. It is also important to note that adolescents of color have lower abortion rates than Caucasians do. However, according to studies released in 2003 by The Alan Guttmacher Institute, those trends are changing, as African American teens are having abortions at a higher rate than they were ten years ago.

Will this trend help bring down the disproportionately high birth rates among African American and Latina teens? If so, it will not be a victory for successful teenage pregnancy prevention initiatives. While some of these teens do not succumb to what Levine calls *compulsory motherhood*—they are not exercising the healthiest decision possible: to prevent an unwanted pregnancy in the first place.

Recent reports highlighting the decline in the number of teen births is cause for celebration. But our work will not be finished until young people have consistent access to all the information, contraception and health services they need to avoid unwanted pregnancy and sexually transmitted disease and ultimately live happy, healthy lives.

Endnotes

Introduction
1. *No Time for Complacency: Teen Births in California.* Public Health Institute, Center for Research on Adolescent Health and Development, Constantine NA & Nevarez CR, 2003.
2. Family Planning Perspectives, 1998.

Chapter 2
1. Darrock and Singh, 1999.
2. Martin, Park et al., 2002.
3. Alan Guttmacher Institute, 2001.
4. California Department of Health Services, n.d.
5. California Department of Health Services, n.d.
6. Clayton, Brindis et al., 2000.
9. Cooksey, 1990.
8. Berglas, Brindis, Cohen, 2003.
9. Brindis & Jeremy, 1988.
10. Clayton, Brindis et al., 2000.
11. Clayton, Brindis et al., 2000.
12. Berglas, Brindis, Cohen, 2003.
13. Brindis & Dearney, 2000.
14. Berglas, Brindis, Cohen, 2003.
15. Clayton, Brindis et al., 2000.

Chapter 3 – Sarah Brown
1. *Not Just Another Single Issue: Teen Pregnancy Prevention's Link*

to Other Critical Social Issues. Washington, D.C.: Author, National Campaign to Prevent Teen Pregnancy, 2002.
2. *With One Voice: America's Adults and Teens Sound Off About Teen Pregnancy.* Washington, D.C.: Author, National Campaign to Prevent Teen Pregnancy (2001-2003).
3. *Do Adolescents Want Babies? The Relationship Between Attitudes and Behavior. Journal of Research on Adolescence,* 3(1), 67-68, Zabin LS, Astone NM & Emerson MR, 1993.
4. *With One Voice: America's Adults and Teens Sound Off About Teen Pregnancy. National Campaign to Prevent Teen Pregnancy,* Washington, D.C., 2001.
5. *Emerging Answers: Research Findings on Programs to Reduce Teen Pregnancy.* Washington, D.C.: The National Campaign to Prevent Teen Pregnancy, Kirby D, 2001.
6. *Promising the Future: Virginity Pledges and the Transition to First Intercourse. American Journal of Sociology,* 106 (4), 859-912, Bearman PS, Bruckner H, 2001.
7. *Halfway There: A Prescription for Continued Progress in Preventing Teen Pregnancy. National Campaign to Prevent Teen Pregnancy,* Washington, D.C., 2001.
8. *A Statistical Portrait of Adolescent Sex, Contraception and Childbearing.* Moore KA, Driscoll AK & Lindberg LD, 1998.
9. *Parent Power: What Parents Need to Know and Do to Help Prevent Teen Pregnancy.* Washington, D.C.: Author. National Campaign to Prevent Teen Pregnancy, 2003.
10. *Reducing the Risk: Connections that Make a Difference in the Lives of Youth.* Minneapolis, MN: University of Minnesota, Center for Adolescent Health and Development, Blum RW, & Rinehart PM, 1998.
11. *Sex Education in America: A View from Inside the Nation's Classrooms.* Menlo Park, CA: Author, The Kaiser Family Foundation, 2000.
12. *14 and Younger: The Sexual Behavior of Young Adolescents.* Washington, D.C.: National Campaign to Prevent Teen Pregnancy, Albert B, Brown S & Flanigan C (Eds.), 2003.
13. *Ibid.*

14. *Talking Back: What Teens Want Adults to Know About Teen Pregnancy.* Washington, D.C.: Author, National Campaign to Prevent Teen Pregnancy, 2003.

Chapter 4 – Susan Philliber, Ph.D.
1. For example, Advocates for Youth. *Science and Success: Sex Education and Other Programs that Work to Prevent Teen Pregnancy, HIV & Sexually Transmitted Infections.* Washington, D.C.: Advocates for Youth, 2003. *Teen Risk-Taking: Promising Prevention Programs and Approaches.* Washington, D.C.: The Urban Institute, Eisen M, Pallitto C, Bradner C & Bolshun N, 2000; *Emerging Answers: Research Findings to Reduce Teen Pregnancy.* Washington, D.C.: The National Campaign to Prevent Teen Pregnancy, Kirby D, 2001.

Chapter 5 – Douglas Kirby, Ph.D.
1. *Emerging Answers: Research Findings on Programs to Reduce Teen Pregnancy,* Kirby, 2001.
2. *Abstinence and Safer Sex: A Randomized Trial of HIV Sexual Risk-Reduction Interventions for Young African-American Adolescents. Journal of the American Medical Association,* 279 (19): 1529-1536, Jemmott, Jemmott & Fong, 1998; *Reducing the Risk: A New Curriculum to Prevent Sexual Risk-Taking. Family Planning Perspectives,* 23 (6):253-263, Kirby, Barth, Leland & Fetro, 1991; *Cognitive Behavioral Intervention to Reduce African American Adolescents' Risk for HIV Infection. Journal of Consulting and Clinical Psychology,* 63(2):221-237, St. Lawrence JS, Brasfield TL, Jefferson KW, Alleyne E, O'Bannon III RE, Shirley A, 1995; *Reducing STD and HIV Risk Behavior of Substance-Dependent Adolescents: A Randomized Controlled Trial. Journal of Consulting and Clinical Psychology* 70(4):1010-1021, St. Lawrence JS, Crosby RA, Brasfield TL and O'Bannon III RE, 2002; *A Randomized, Controlled Effectiveness Trial of an AIDS Prevention Program for Low-Income African-American*

Youths. Archives of *Pediatric Adolescent Medicine* 150:363-372, Stanton BF, Li X, Ricardo I, Galbraith J, Feigelman S & Kaljee L, 1996.

3. *Safer Choices: Reducing Teen Pregnancy, HIV and STDs.* Public Health Reports, Supplement 1, 116: 82-93, Coyle KK, Basen-Engquist KM, Kirby DB, Parcel GS, Banspack SW, Collins JL, Baumler ER, Carvajal S, Harrist RB, 2001.

4. *Safer Choices: Reducing Teen Pregnancy, HIV and STDs.* Public Health Reports, Supplement 1, 116: 82-93, Coyle et al., 2001; *Abstinence and Safer Sex: A Randomized Trial of HIV Sexual Risk-Reducation Interventions for Young African-American Adolescents. Journal of the American Medical Association,* 279 (19): 1529-1536, Jemmott, Jemmott & Fong, 1998; *Cognitive Behavioral Intervention to Reduce African American Adolescents' Risk for HIV Infection. Journal of Consulting and Clinical Psychology,* 63(2):221-23, St. Lawrence et al., 1995.

5. *HIV Risk Reduction Behavioral Interventions with Heterosexual Adolescents.* AIDS 14 (SUPPL 2): s40-s52, Jemmott & Jemmott, 2000; *Emerging Answers: Research Findings on Programs to Reduce Teen Pregnancy,* Kirby, 2001; *Meta-Analysis of the Effects of Behavioral HIV Prevention Interventions on the Sexual Risk Behavior of Sexually Experienced Adolescents in Controlled Studies in the United States. Journal of Acquired Immune Deficiency Syndromes* 30:S94-S105, Mullen, Ramirez, Strouse, Hedges & Sogolow, 2002.

6. c.f. *HIV Risk Reducation Behavioral Interventions with Heterosexual Adolescents.* AIDS 14 (SUPPL 2):s40-s52, Jemmott & Jemmott, 2000; *Emerging Answers: Research Findings on Programs to Reduce Teen Pregnancy,* Kirby, 2001.

7. Allen, Philliber, Herrling & Kuperminc, 1997; *National Evaluation of Learn and Serve America School and Community-Based Programs.* Waltham, MA, Center for Human Resources, Brandeis University, Melchior, 1998; *The Effectiveness of the Reach for Health Community Youth Service Learning Program in Reducing Early and Unprotected Sex*

Among Urban Middle School Students. *American Journal of Public Health* 89(2):176-181, O'Donnell L, Stueve A, Doval AS et al, 1999; *Long-Term Reducations in Sexual Initiation and Sexual Activity Among Urban Middle Schoolers in the Reach for Health Service Learning Program.* Journal of Adolescent Health 31:93-100, O'Donnell et al, 2002; Life Options and Community Service: Teen Outreach Program. In Miller BC, Card JJ, Paikoff RL and Peterson JL (eds). *Preventing Adolescent Pregnancy.* Newbury Park: Sage Publications, Philliber & Allen, 1992.

8. Philliber et al., 2002.
9. *Get Organized: A Guide to Preventing Teen Pregnancy.* Washington, D.C.: National Campaign to Prevent Teen Pregnancy, Kreinin T, Khun S, Rodgers AB & Hutchins J, 1999.
10. c.f. *Logic Models: A Useful Tool for Designing, Stregthening and Evaluating Programs to Reduce Adolescent Sexual Risktaking, Pregnancy, HIV and Other STDs.* Scotts Valley, CA: ETR Associates, Kirby, 2003.

Chapter 6 – Voices of California Adaptation

1. California State Census Data, 2000.
2. California Department of Health Services, 2002.
3. California Department of Health Services, 2002.
4. *A Community Dialogue on Teen Pregnancy Prevention Among Southeast Asians.* The Get Real About Teen Pregnancy Campaign.
5. The Sacramento Bee, Dec. 2002.
6. California Department of Health Services, 2002.
7. Clayton SL, Brindis CD, Hamor JA, Raiden-Wright H, Fong C. *Investing in Adolescent Health: A Social Imperative for California's Future.* San Francisco: University of California, San Francisco, National Adolescent Health Information Center, January, 2001.
8. Youth Risk Behavior Surveillance, 1999.
9. U.S. Census Data 2000.

10. Fact Sheet on *Latino Youth: Sexual Behavior*, Center for Reproductive Health Research and Policy, 2002.
11. U.S. Census Data 2000.
12. Fact Sheet on *Latino Youth: Sexual Behavior*, Institute for Health Policy Studies, 2001.
13. California Center for Health Statistics, 2002.
14. California Department of Health Services, Office of Family Planning, 1999.
15. Driscoll AK, Biggs MA, Brindis CD, Yankah E, *Adolescent Latino Reproductive Health: A Review of Literature. Hispanic Journal of the Behavioral Sciences,* 2001 Oct, 23(3): 255-326.
16. *Adolescent Latino Reproductive Health: A Review of the Literature,* Institute for Health Policy Studies, 2001.
17. Ibid.

Chapter 9 – Kathy Kneer
1. Abbott 2000; D'Emilio & Freedman, 1998: McLauren, 1990.
2. Brandt, 1985; Bullough & Bullogh, 1987.

Chapter 11 – Cynthia Dailard
1. Northern Kentucky University, Lipsitz A, 2003.
2. *Virginity and the First Time.* Kaiser Family Foundation, Seventeen Magazine, 2003.
3. Northern Kentucky University, Lipsitz A, 2003.

Chapter 12 – Tom Klaus
1. Family Planning Perspectives, Volume 31, No. 2, March/April 1999.
2. Health Education and Behavior, 26, 1999, 43-54.

Chapter 14 – Rev. Debra W. Haffner
1. *A Time To Speak. NY: SIECUS, Haffner DW, 1998.*
2. *Faithful Nation. National Campaign To Prevent Teenage Pregnancy.*
3. *Risky Sex Less Likely for Religious Teens, Reuters Health news release, October 29, 2001.*

4. *Faithful Nation. National Campaign.*
5. *Faith Matters. Christian Community.*
6. *Faith Matters. Christian Community.*
7. *Faithful Nation. National Campaign.*
8. *Faith Matters. Christian Community.*
9. *Faithful Nation. National Campaign.*
10. *Faith Matters. Christian Community.*
11. *Faith Matters. Christian Community.*
12. *Faithful Nation. National Campaign.*
13. *A Time To Speak.* NY: SIECUS, Haffner, DW, 1998.
14. *An Open Letter to Religious Educators on Sex Education, op. cit.*
15. This list is used with permission from D.W. Haffner, *A Time To Build: Creating Sexually Healthy Faith Communities.* (Connecticut: Religious Institute, 2002).

Chapter 16 – Barbara Staggers, M.D.

1. *Adolescent Sexuality at the dawn of the 21st century.* Adolescent Medicine, Brown RT, 2000;11:19; BrooksGunn J, Furstenburg FF J. *Adolescent Sexual Behavior.* Am Psychol 44: 249, 1989; Adolescent Sexuality in Hoekelman R et al. Eds. Primary Pediatric Care. St. Lois: Mosby–Year Book, Inc., Coupey S, 1997; <u>*Facing Facts: Sexual Health of America's Adolescents*</u>. The Report of the National Commission on Adolescent Sexual Health. Debra Haffner, editor. Copyright 1995; *National Survey of Adolescents and Young Adults: Sexual Health Knowledge, Attitude, and Experiences,* Hoff T, et al. Menlo Park, CA: Henry Kaiser Family Foundation, 2003; *(Making the Connection) Definitions of Sexually Related Health Terminology.* The Sexuality Information and Education Council of the U.S. (SIECUS) 1999.
2. <u>*Facing Facts: Sexual Health of America's Adolescents.*</u> The Report of the National Commission on Adolescent Sexual Health. Debra Haffner, editor. Copyright 1995.
3. Adolescent Health Care: A Practical Guide (Philadelphia) Neinstein, LS, Lippincott, Williams, and Wilkins. 2002.

4. *Childhood and adolescent sexuality.* Pediatr Clin North Am, Duncan P, Dixon RR, Carison J, 2003-9-11 50(4)765–80; *Promoting Healthy Sexual Development During Early Adolescence.* In: Lerner RM(Ed). Early Adolescent Perspectives on research, policy, and intervention. New York: Erl Baun, Koch PB, 1993: 293 – 307.
5. *Childhood and adolescent sexuality.* Pediatric Clinic North America, Duncan P,Dixon RR, Carison J, 2003-9-11 50(4)765–80.
6. Conceptual identity: establish and place oneself within religious, cultural, moral and political environmental constructs.
7. Functional identity: preparing oneself for adult roles in society by identifying competencies.
8. Sexual self-concept: experience of adult-like erotic feeling, experimentation and sense of gender identity/orientation.
9. <u>*Facing Facts: Sexual Health of America's Adolescents.*</u> The Report of the National Commission on Adolescent Sexual Health. Debra Haffner, editor. Copyright 1995.
10. Adolescent Health Care: A Practical Guide. (Philadelphia), Neinstein, LS, Lippincott, Williams, and Wilkins. 2002.
11. <u>*Facing Facts: Sexual Health of America's Adolescents.*</u> The Report of the National Commission on Adolescent Sexual Health. Debra Haffner, editor. Copyright 1995.
12. *Adolescent Sexuality* in Hoekelman R et al. Eds. Priimary Pediatric Care. St. Lois: Mosby – Year Book, Inc., Coupey S., 1997; <u>*Facing Facts: Sexual Health of America's Adolescents.*</u> The Report of the National Commission on Adolescent Sexual Health. Debra Haffner, editor. Copyright 1995; Adolescent Health Care: A Practical Guide. (Philadelphia), Neinstein, LS, Lippincott, Williams, and Wilkins. 2002.
13. *Teenage pregnancy: overall trends and state-by-state information,* Alan Guttmacher Institute,. New York: AGI, 1999;

Adolescent Sexuality at the dawn of the 21st century. Adolesc Med, Brown RT, 2000;11:19; *Adolescent Sexual Behavior,* BrooksGunn J, Furstenburg FF J. Am Psychol 44: 249 , 1989; *Facing Facts: Sexual Health of America's Adolescents.* The Report of the National Commission on Adolescent Sexual Health. Debra Haffner, editor. Copyright 1995; *Fourteen and Younger: The Sexual behavior of Young Adolescents.* Washington, D.C.: The National Campaign to Prevent Teen Pregnancy, 2003; *AIDS–Related Risk Among Adolescent Males Who Have Sex with Males, Females, or Both: Evidence from a Statewide Survey.* American Journal of Public Health, Goodenow, C. et al, February 2002, vol. 92, no. 2, pp. 203 – 9; *"Youth Risk Behavior Surveillance (YRBS)- United States,* Grumbaun, J., et al, 2001; Morbidity and Mortality Weekly Report, vol. 51, no. SS-4, June 28, 2002, pp 1- 64; *National Survey of Adolescents and Young Adults: Sexual Health Knowledge, Attitude, and Experiences.* Menlo Park, CA: Henry Kaiser Family Foundation, Hoff, T., et al., 2003; *"Youth Risk Behavior Surveillance, 1995. Surveillance Summarie,"* Kann, Laura, PhD., et al., September 27, 1996. Morbidity and Mortality Weekly Support, 1996: vol. 45, no SS –4 pp 1–83; *Health, United States, 2000: Adolescent Health Chartbook* (Hyattsville MD: National Center for Health Statistics, 2000; *The Truth About Adolescent Sexuality.* The Sexuality Information and Education Council of the U.S. (SIECUS) Fact Sheet, MacKay AP, Fingerhut LA, Duran CR, Fall 2003.
14. *"Youth Risk Behavior Surveillance (YRBS)–United States,* 2001; Morbidity and Mortality Weekly Report, Grumbaun, J., et al., vol. 51, no. SS-4, June 28, 2002, pp 1- 64.
15. Alan Guttmacher Institute, *In Their Own Right: Addressing the Sexual and Reproductive Health Needs of American Men.* New York: AGI, 2002; American Academy of Pediatrics, *Homosexuality and Adolescents. Pediatrics,* 1993;92(4); 631–34; *Adolescent homosexuality: we need to learn more about causes and consequences,* Acta Paediatr., Berg–Kelly K,

2003;92(2):141 – 4; *Sexual identity development among sexual-minoity male youths.* Dev Psychol, Dube EM, Savin_Williams RC, 1999;35(6):1389–1398; AIDS–*Related Risk Among Adolescent Males Who Have Sex with Males, Females, or Both: Evidence from a Statewide Survey.* American Journal of Public Health, Goodenow, C. et al, February 2002, vol. 92, no. 2, pp. 203–9; *Primary Care of lesbian and gay patients: educating ourselves and our students.* Family Medicine, Harrison AE, 1996;28:10–23; *(Making the Connection) Definitions of Sexually Related Health Terminology.* The Sexuality Information and Education Council of the U.S. (SIECUS) 1999; *Adolescent Homosexuality. Psychosocial and medical implications.* Pediatrics 79:331–37, Remafedi, G, 1987; *Lesbian and Gay youth: Care and Counseling.* NY: Columbia University Press, Ryan C and Futterman D, 1998; *Sexuality Orientation and Identity.* The Sexuality Information and Education Council of the U.S. (SIECUS) Fact Sheet, 2003; *Sexual Intercourse, Abuse and Pregnancy Among Adolescent Women: Does sexual Orientation Make a Difference?* Family Planning Perspectives. 199, vol. 31, no. 3, pp. 127–31; Stronski–Hawiler SM, Remafedi G. *Adolescent Homosexuality.* Advances in Pediatrics, Saewyc, E.M., et al., 1998; 45:107–45; *Homosexual Identity Development.* Journal of Adolescent Health Care, Troiden RR, 1998; 9:105–113.

16. Homosexual Identity Development. Journal of Adolescent Health Care, Troiden RR, 1998; 9:105-113.
17. Sexual Identity Development Among Sexual-Minority Male Youths. Developmental Psychology, Dube EM, Savin, Williams RC, 1999; 35(6):1389–1398.
18. Adolescent Homosexuality. Advances in Pediatrics, Stronski–Hawiler SM, Remafedi G, 1998; 45:107–45.
19. Primary Care of Lesbian and Gay Patients: Educating Ourselves and Our Students. Family Medicine, Harrison AE, 1996;28:10–23.

Chapter 17 – Barbara Huberman
1. *Trends in pregnancy rates for the United States, 1976-97: an update.* National Vital Statistics Reports, Ventura SJ et al., 2001;49(4):1-10.
2. Calculations based on Feijoo, AN. *Teenage Pregnancy, the Case for Prevention.* Washington D.C.: Advocates for Youth, 1999.
3. *Sex Education in the Netherlands.* Paper presented to the European Study Tour. Leiden, Netherlands:NISSO, Rademakers J, 2001.
4. *Births: preliminary data for 2000.* National Vital Statistics Reports Martin, JA et al., 2001;49(5):1-20.
5. *Sexually transmitted diseases among adolescents in developed countries.* Family Planning Perspectives, Panchaud, C. et al., 2000;32(1):24-32&45.
6. *Adolescent Sexual and Reproductive Health: A Developed Country Comparison.* New York, NY: Darroch, JE et al. The Alan Guttmacher Institute, forthcoming.

Additional References:

Allen, J. P., & Philliber, S. P. (2001). *Who Benefits Most From a Broadly Targeted Prevention Program?: Differential Efficacy Across Populations in the Teen Outreach Program.* Journal of Community Psychology, 29, 637-655.

Allen, J.P., Philliber, S., & Hoggson, N. (1990). *School-based Prevention of Teen-age Pregnancy and School Dropout: Process Evaluation of the National Replication of the Teen Outreach Program.* American Journal of Community Psychology, 18(4), 505-524.

Barth RP. *Reducing the Risk: Building Skills to Prevent Pregnancy, STD & HIV.* Santa Cruz, CA: ETR Publications, 3rd edition, 1996.

Boekeloo BO, Schamus LA, Simmens SJ, Cheng TL, O'Connor K, D'Angelo LJ. *A STD/HIV Prevention Trial*

Among Adolescents in Managed Care. Pediatrics 103(1): 107-115, 1999.

Bickel, R., Weaver, S., Williams, T., & Lange, L. (1997.) *Opportunity, Community, and Teen Pregnancy in an Appalachian State.* Journal of Educational Research, 90(3), 175-181.

Billy, J.O.G., Brewster, K.L., & Grady, W.R. (1994). *Contextual Effects on the Sexual Behavior of Adolescent Women.* Journal of Marriage and the Family, 56(2), 387-404.

Brooks-Gunn, J., Duncan, G.J., Klebanov, P.K., & Sealand, N. (1993). *Do Neighborhoods Influence Child and Adolescent Development?* American Journal of Sociology, 99(2), 353-395.

Cornerstone Consulting Group, Inc. *Changing Scenes: A Curriculum of the Teen Outreach Program.* Houston, Cornerstone Consulting Group, Inc. 2002.

Coyle KK and Fetro JV. *Safer Choices: Preventing HIV, Other STD and Pregnancy: Level 2.* Santa Cruz, Calif.: ETR Associates, 1998.

Coyle KK, Basen-Engquist KM, Kirby, Parcel GS, Banspach SW, Collins JL, Baumler ER, Carvajal S, Harrist RB. *Safer Choices: Reducing Teen Pregnancy, HIV and STDs. Public Health Reports,* Supplement 1, 116: 82-93, 2001.

Coyle K, Marin B, Gardner C, et al., *Draw the Line: Respect the Line: Setting Limits to Prevent HIV, STD and Pregnancy. Grade 7.* Scotts Valley, California: ETR Associates. 2003.

Coyle K, Kirby D, Marin B, Gomez C, Gregorich S. *Draw the Line/Respect the Line: A Randomized Trial of a Middle School Intervention to Reduce Sexual Risk Behaviors.* Submitted for review.

Danielson R, Marcy S, Plunkett A, Wiest W and Greenlick MR. *Reproductive Health Counseling for Young Men: What Does It Do? Family Planning Perspectives,* 22(3):115 121, May/June, 1990.

Ekstrand ML, Siegel D, Nido V, Faigeles B, Cummings G, Battle R, Krasnovsky F, Chiment E, Coates TJ. *Peer-led AIDS*

Prevention Delays Onset of Sexual Activity and Changes Peer Norms Among Urban Junior High School Students. Journal of Acquired Immune Deficiency Syndromes and Human Retrovirology, in press.

Fetro JV, Barth RB and Coyle KK. *Safer Choices: Preventing HIV, Other STD and Pregnancy: Level 1.* Santa Cruz, Calif.: ETR Associate, 1998.

Fisher JD. *Possible effects of reference group-based social influence on AIDS-risk behaviors and AIDS.* American Psychologist, 43:914-920, 1988.

Grunbaum JA, Kann L, Kinchen SA, Williams B, Ross JG, Lowry R, Kolbe L. *Youth risk behavior surveillance — United States, 2001.* In: Surveillance Summaries, June 28, 2002. MMWR 2002; 51 (No.SS-4):48.

Henshaw SK. *Unintended Pregnancy in the United States. Family Planning Perspectives* 30(1), 24-29, 42, 1998.

Henshaw SK. U.S. *Teenage Pregnancy Statistics with Comparative Statistics for Women Aged 20-24.* New York: The Alan Guttmacher Institute, 2001.

Hogan, D.P., & Kitagawa, E.M. (1985). *The Impact of Social Status, Family Structure, and Neighborhood on the Fertility of Black Adolescents.* American Journal of Sociology, 90(4), 825-855.

Howard M, Mitchel M and Pollard B. *Postponing Sexual Involvement: An Educational Series for Young Teens.* Atlanta: Grady Memorial Hospital, 1990.

Jemmott LS, Jemmott III JB and McCaffree KA. *Be Proud! Be Responsible!* New York: Select Media, 1994.

Jemmott JB, Jemmott LS, and Fong GT. *Abstinence and Safer Sex: A Randomized Trial of HIV Sexual Risk-reduction Interventions for Young African-American Adolescents.* Journal of the American Medical Association, 279(19): 1529-1536, 1998.

Jemmott LS and Jemmott JB: Making Proud Choices: *A Safer Sex Approach to STD, Teen Pregnancy and HIV/AIDS Prevention.* Select Media, 1998/9.

Jemmott JB and Jemmott LS. *HIV Risk Reduction Behavioral Interventions with Heterosexual Adolescents*. AIDS 14 (SUPPL 2):s40-s52, 2000.

Jemmott LS and Jemmott JB: Making A Difference: *An Abstinence Approach to STD, Teen Pregnancy and HIV/AIDS Prevention*. Select Media, 1998/9.

Kirby D. *Emerging Answers: Research Findings on Programs to Reduce Sexual Risk-Taking and Teen Pregnancy*. Washington D.C.: National Campaign to Prevent Teen Pregnancy, 2001.

Kirby D. Logic models: *A Useful Tool for Designing, Strengthening and Evaluating Programs to Reduce Adolescent Sexual Risk-taking, Pregnancy,* HIV and other STDs. Scotts Valley, CA: ETR Associates, 2003.

Kirby D, Barth R, Leland N and Fetro J. *Reducing the Risk: A New Curriculum to Prevent Sexual Risk-taking*. Family Planning Perspectives, 23(6):253-263, 1991.

Kirby D, Coyle K, Gould J. *Manifestations of Poverty and Birth Rates Among Young Teenagers in California ZIP codes*. Family Planning Perspectives. 33(2):63-69, 2001.

Klaus H, Bryan LM, Bryant ML et al., *Fertility Awareness/Natural Family Planning for Adolescents and their Families: Report of a Multisite Pilot Project*. International Journal of Adolescent Medicine and Health 3(2): 101-119, 1987

Kreinin T, Kuhn S, Rodgers AB, & Hutchins J. (Eds.). *Get Organized: A Guide to Preventing Teen Pregnancy*. Washington, D.C.: National Campaign to Prevent Teen Pregnancy, 1999.

Ku, L., Sonenstein, F.L., & Pleck, J.H. (1993). *Neighborhood, Family, and Work: Influences on the Premarital Behaviors of Adolescent Males*. Social Forces, 72(2), 479-503.

Magura S, Kang S and Shapiro JL. *Outcomes of Intensive AIDS Education for Male Adolescent Drug Users in Jail*. Journal of Adolescent Health, 15:457-463, 1994.

Main DS, Iverson DC, McGloin J, Banspach SW, Collins K, Rugg D and Kolbe LJ. *Preventing HIV Infection Among Adolescents: Evaluation of a School-based Education Program.* Preventing Medicine, 23:409-417, 1994.

Marin B, Coyle K, Gomez C, et al., *Draw the Line: Respect the Line: Setting Limits to Prevent HIV, STD and Pregnancy. Grade 6.* Scotts Valley, California: ETR Associates. 2003.

Marin B, Coyle K, Cummings C, et al., *Draw the Line: Respect the Line: Setting Limits to Prevent HIV, STD and Pregnancy. Grade 8.* Scotts Valley, California: ETR Associates. 2003.

Martin JA, Park MM, Sutton PD. Births: Preliminary data for 2001. *National Vital Statistics Reports* 50(10). Hyattsville, M.D., 2002.

Mayer, S.E., & Jencks, C. (1989). *Growing up in poor neighborhoods: How much does it matter?* Science, 243(4897), 1441-1445.

Melchior, A. (1998). *National evaluation of Learn and Serve America School and Community-based Programs.* Waltham, MA: Center for Human Resources, Brandeis University.

Moore, K. A. & Ooms, T. (1997). *Not Just for Girls: The Role of Boys and Men in Teen Pregnancy Prevention.* Washington, D.C.: National Campaign to Prevent Teen Pregnancy.

Mullen PD, Ramirez G, Strouse D, Hedges LV and Sogolow E. *Meta-analysis of the Effects of Behavioral HIV Prevention Interventions on the Sexual Risk Behavior of Sexually Experienced Adolescents in Controlled Studies in the United States.* Journal of Acquired Immune Deficiency Syndromes 30: S94-S105, 2002.

National Campaign to Prevent Teen Pregnancy. *Whatever Happened to Childhood? The Problem of Teen Pregnancy in the United States.* Washington, D.C.: National Campaign to Prevent Teen Pregnancy, 1997.

O'Donnell L, Stueve A, Doval AS et al. *The Effectiveness of the Reach for Health Community Youth Service Learning Program in Reducing Early and Unprotected Sex Among Urban Middle School Students.* American Journal of Public Health 89(2):176-181, 1999.

O'Donnell L, Stueve A, O'Donnel C, Duran R, Doval AS, Wilson RF, Haber D, Perry E, Pleck JH. *Long-term Reductions in Sexual Initiation and Sexual Activity Among Urban Middle Schoolers in the Reach for Health Service Learning Program.* Journal of Adolescent Health 31:93-100, 2002.

Orr, D.P., Langefeld, C.D., Katz, B.P., & Caine, V.A. (1996). *Behavioral Intervention to Increase Condom use Among High-risk Female Adolescents.* Journal of Pediatrics, 128(2), 288-295.

Philliber S and Allen JP. *Life Options and Community Service: Teen Outreach Program.* In Miller BC, Card JJ, Paikoff RL and Peterson JL (eds). *Preventing Adolescent Pregnancy.* Newbury Park: Sage Publications, 1992.

Rotheram-Borus MJ, Koopman C, Haigners C and Davies M. *Reducing HIV Sexual Risk Behaviors Among Runaway Adolescents.* Journal of the American Medical Association, 266(9): 1237-1241, September 4, 1991.

Sonenstein, F. et. al. (1997). *Involving Males in Teen Pregnancy Prevention: A Guide for Program Planners.* Washington, D.C.: The Urban Institute.

St. Lawrence JS. *Becoming a Responsible Teen: An HIV Risk Reduction Intervention for African-American Adolescents.* Scotts Valley, CA: ETR Associates, 1998.

St. Lawrence JS, Brasfield TL, Jefferson KW, Alleyne E, O'Bannon III RE, Shirley A. *Cognitive-Behavioral Intervention to Reduce African American Adolescents' Risk for HIV infection.* Journal of Consulting and Clinical Psychology, 63(2):221-237, 1995.

St. Lawrence JS, Crosby RA, Brasfield TL and O'Bannon III RE. *Reducing STD and HIV risk Behavior of Substance-dependent Adolescents: A Randomized Controlled Trial.* Journal of Consulting and Clinical Psychology 70(4):1010-1021, 2002.

Stanton BF, Li X, Ricardo I, Galbraith J, Feigelman S and Kaljee L. *A Randomized, Controlled Effectiveness Trial of an AIDS Prevention Program for Low-income African-American Youths.* Archives of Pediatric Adolescent Medicine 150:363-372, 1996.

Sylvester K. & Reich. K. (2002). *Making Fathers Count: Assessing the Progress of Responsible Fatherhood Efforts.* Washington, D.C.: Social Policy Action Network.

Thomas B, Mitchell A, Devlin M, Goldsmith C, Singer J and Watters D. *Small Group Sex Education at School: the McMaster Teen Program.* In Miller B, Card J, Paikoff R, Peterson J: *Preventing Adolescent Pregnancy.* Newbury Park, CA: Sage Publications, 28-52, 1992.

Ventura SJ, Mosher WD, Curtin SC, Abma JC, *Trends in Pregnancy Rates for the United States, 1976-97: An Update.* National vital statistics reports: vol 49(4). Hyattsville, M.D.: National Center for Health Statistics, 2001.

Walter HJ and Vaughn RD. *AIDS Risk Reduction Among a Multi-ethnic Sample of Urban High School Students.* Journal of the American Medical Association, 270(6): 725-730, 1993.

Winter L and Breckenmaker LC. *Tailoring Family Planning Services to the Special Needs of Adolescents.* Family Planning Perspectives, 23(1):24-30, January/February, 1991.

In Their Own Right: Addressing the Sexual and Reproductive Health Needs of American Men (2002). New York, NY: The Alan Guttmacher Institute.

Innovative Approaches to Increase Parent-Child Communication about Sexuality: Their Impact and Examples from the Field (2002). New York, NY: Sexuality Information and Education Council of the United States (SIECUS).

Young Men Moving Forward: California's Male Involvement Program, a Teen Pregnancy Prevention Program for Males (2002). Sacramento CA: California Department of Health Services, Office of Family Planning.